EAT BUT
DON'T
PIG OUT

EAT BUT DON'T PIG OUT

THE RIGHT WAY TO EAT AND HEAL YOUR BODY

LIGHT WALKER

AKA Kd Royal who is known as Kaliq Menkuare El

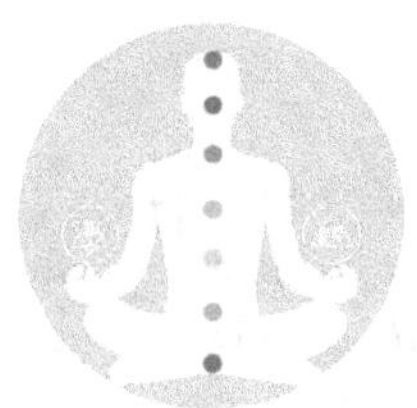

Eat But Don't Pig Out
Light Walker

CONTENTS

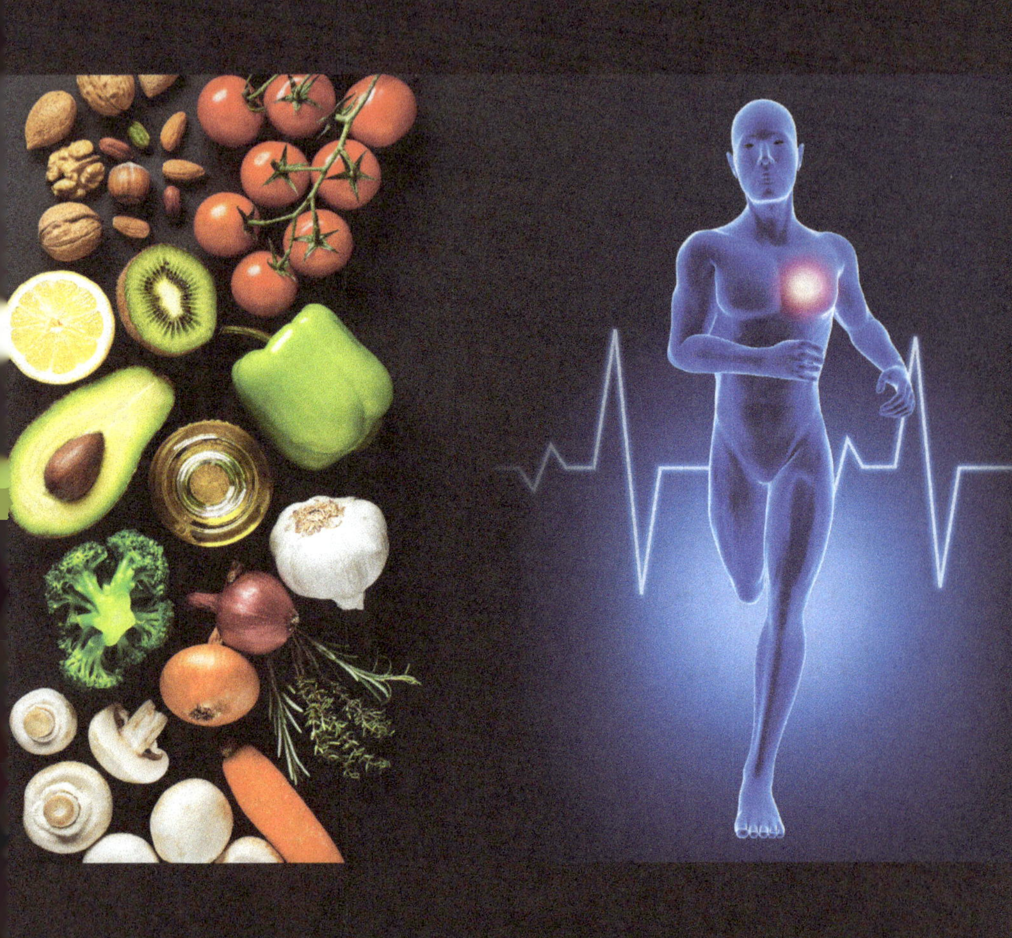

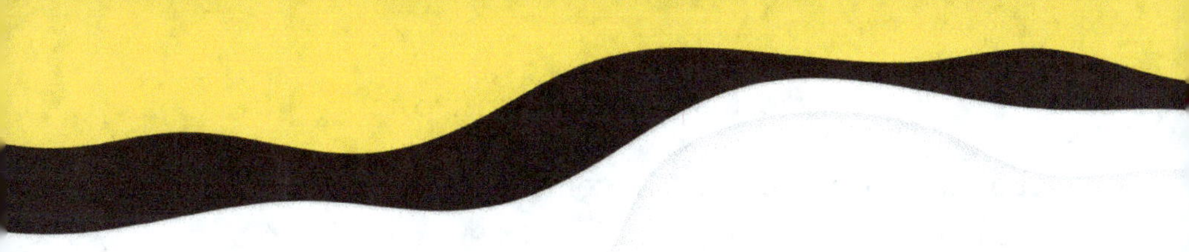

One thing that I notice from being born and raised in the western society is that the people have a strong desire to consume pork. They must break away from this programming in order to live most healthy and prosperous lives that the Most High intended for us to have.

Genesis 1:29
And God said, Behold, I have given you every herb bearing seed, which is upon the face of all the earth, and every tree, in the which is the fruit of a tree yielding seed; to you it shall be for meat.

Many believe and assume that Followers of Judaism and Islam are forbidden from eating pork but I find it strange that Christianity also mention to its followers that pork shall not be eating.

Leviticus 11:7-8
And the pig, because it parts the hoof and is cloven-footed but does not chew the cud, is unclean to you. You shall not eat any of their flesh, and you shall not touch their carcasses; they are unclean to you.

Isaiah 66:17
"Those who sanctify and purify themselves to go into the gardens, following one in the midst, eating pig's flesh and the

abomination and mice, shall come to an end together, declares the Lord.

Deuteronomy 14:8
And the pig, because it parts the hoof but does not chew the cud, is unclean for you. Their flesh you shall not eat, and their carcasses you shall not touch

The Bible says that He will give us more life abundantly, but He demands strict obedience to His Will
The Foods that we consume play a major role in our health

Leading Causes of Death
Data are for the U.S.
Number of deaths for leading causes of death

- Heart disease: 696,962
- Cancer: 602,350
- COVID-19: 350,831
- Accidents (unintentional injuries): 200,955
- Stroke (cerebrovascular diseases): 160,264
- Chronic lower respiratory diseases: 152,657
- Alzheimer's disease: 134,242
- Diabetes: 102,188
- Influenza and pneumonia: 53,544
- Nephritis, nephrotic syndrome, and nephrosis: 52,547

The number 1 killer amongst not just my people but the world is heart disease.

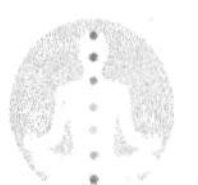

HEART DISEASE

Heart and blood vessel disease (also called heart disease) includes numerous problems, many of which are related to a process called atherosclerosis.

Atherosclerosis is a condition that develops when a substance called plaque builds up in the walls of the arteries. This buildup narrows the arteries, making it harder for blood to flow through. If a blood clot forms, it can block the blood flow. This can cause a heart attack or stroke.

Heart attack

A heart attack occurs when the blood flow to a part of the heart is blocked by a blood clot. If this clot cuts off the blood flow completely, the part of the heart muscle supplied by that artery begins to die.

Most people survive their first heart attack and return to their normal lives, enjoying many more years of productive activity. But experiencing a heart attack does mean that you need to make some changes like changing the types of food that you eat .The medications and lifestyle changes that your doctor recommends may vary according to how badly your heart was damaged, and to what degree of heart disease caused the heart attack.

Learn more about heart attack.

Stroke

An ischemic stroke (the most common type of stroke) occurs when a blood vessel that feeds the brain gets blocked, usually from a blood clot.

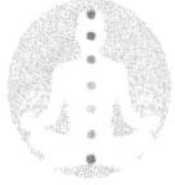

When the blood supply to a part of the brain is cut off, some brain cells will begin to die. This can result in the loss of functions controlled by that part of the brain, such as walking or talking.

A hemorrhagic stroke occurs when a blood vessel within the brain bursts. This is most often caused by uncontrolled hypertension (high blood pressure).

Some effects of stroke are permanent if too many brain cells die after being starved of oxygen. These cells are never replaced.

The good news is that sometimes brain cells don't die during stroke — instead, the damage is temporary. Over time, as injured cells repair themselves, previously impaired function improves. (In other cases, undamaged brain cells nearby may take over for the areas of the brain that were injured.)

Either way, strength may return, speech may get better and memory may improve. This recovery process is what stroke rehabilitation is all about.

When it comes to spotting stroke and getting help, the faster, the better. That's because prompt treatment may make the difference between life and death — or the difference between a full recovery and long-term disability. Use the letters in F.A.S.T to spot a stroke. F is for face drooping. A is for arm weakness. S is for speech difficulty. T is for time to call 911.

How much food is consumed daily in America?
US Food Consumption Totals

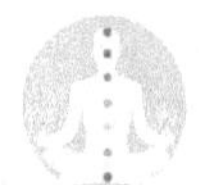

Americans eat 815 billion calories of food each day - that's roughly 200 billion more than needed - enough to feed 80 million people. Americans throw out 200,000 tons of edible food daily. The average American generates 52 tons of garbage by age 75.

If we wish to prolong our lives we must learn to consume the right foods.

Let's pay attention to the facts and the facts are that people are dying more from the foods we eat than from drugs, gang violence and police brutality.

I CAN ONLY HELP YOU IF YOU'RE WILLING TO HELP YOURSELF

Our ancestors who were kidnapped were forced to eat the scraps of the pig with much of nothing and not many other food sources they began to love the swine. The experience was so traumatizing to them that the food was the only form of instant gratification. Now when you look at the elements of the circumstances that our ancestors were subjected to you will overstand that they trauma bonded to the swine and to this very day that is something that is passed down through DNA until we learn to break that cycle.

This is something that is held in our genetic memory. In psychology, genetic memory is a theorized phenomenon in which certain kinds of memories could be inherited.

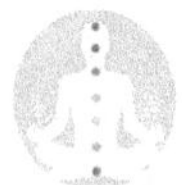

After I look at the current day conditions of my people it is safe to say that we have been attacked with the heavily commercialized food which is mainly pork and we must learn to live without it.

I must say that we have been genetically bred to love pork and to many that may seem far fetched but scientists have confirmed that emotions good or bad, happy or sad can be passed down through the genes. We must learn to detox ourselves and get rid of all of these toxins and poisons that enter our bodies by way of food consumption.

What I now overstand is that my people's condition is so severe concerning this poisonous swine that they may have to undergo therapy because this is a psychological condition for many of us.

There are many foods I wish to teach you not to eat, but so many of you cannot avoid eating them.

We must prepare and grow our own food, because this is a highly commercialized world. They genetically modify a lot of food, and some of this food is not good for our stomachs.

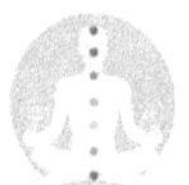

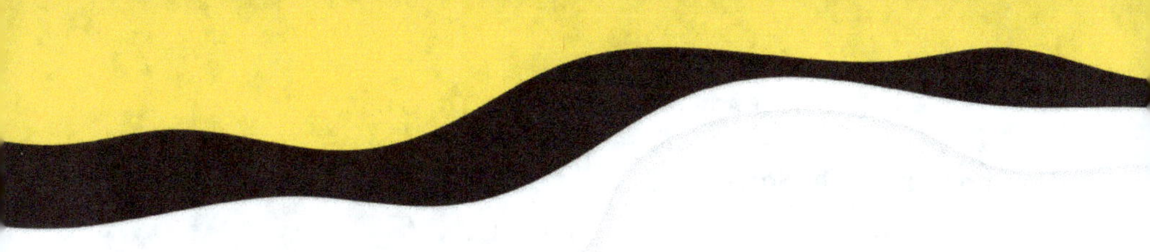

HISTORY ON THE PIG/SWINE

The pig dates back 40 million years to fossils, which indicate that wild pig-like animals roamed forests and swamps in Europe and Asia. By 4900 B.C. pigs were domesticated in China, and were being raised in Europe by 1500 B.C.

The rise of the pig began in Asia and progressed through the Near East, and eventually to Europe, where Sus scrofa domesticus really took off. It is to Spain that the Americas owe the introduction of this valuable animal, as the first pigs on the continent were brought with Columbus on his second voyage. The Spanish explorers brought pigs with them to eat on their long expeditions, and left many of them in the New World, where no large domesticated animals existed. Hernando de Soto, who explored what is today the southeastern United States, is often called the father of the American pork industry, as he brought 200 of them on his expedition. Those that remained are the ancestors of most of the pigs in the country, and certainly related to the feral pigs, or wild boar, that roam the country.

Hernando De Soto

Hernando De Soto, a Spanish explorer, was the first to introduce domestic swine (family Suidae) to the mainland of North America.

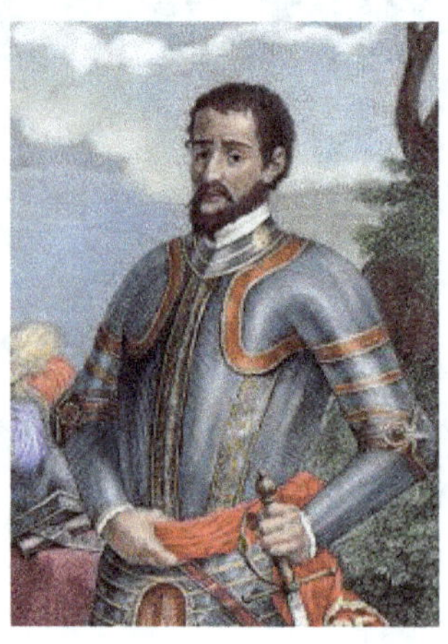

In ancient times certain civilizations like the Egyptians used the pig solemnly what it was created for which was for the purpose of disposing garbage.

From 1872 – 1932 Worcester relied solely on pigs to get rid of the city's garbage. At its height, more than eight thousand pigs were disposing of over 10 tons of garbage a day making it the largest municipal piggery in the country. Due to complaints about the smell and the construction of the city's first garbage incinerator, the piggery was shut down in 1932

Swine is used for other purposes not for a food for the people. Consumption of this animal destroys the beautiful appearance of its eaters.

The pig is complete filth and poison and cannot be poisoned it is a foul animal and lives off nothing but filth.

Snake bites doesn't harm pigs their resistance is to the a-neurotoxin in snake venom, specifically Scientists have discovered that pigs have a genetic mutation in their cell receptors that prevents binding of the a-neurotoxin, rendering the venom useless. The resistance doesn't occur in most pigs until they are adults, so small pigs are still vulnerable.

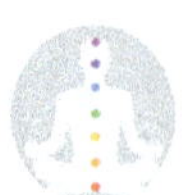

It is true that pigs do not have sweat glands and, therefore, are not able to get rid of toxins in their bodies. On their forelegs is a little hole that releases pus.

Trichinella spiralis is commonly known as "Pork worm" is most common parasite in human infection. The larvae are encapsulated in cysts called "nurse cells" in the muscle tissue of the infected animal and are released upon digestion by pepsin and other digestive enzymes. Once inside the intestine, the nematodes can inhibit the host immune response while they mature, mate and produce more larvae, which then invade muscle tissue in the new host. This initial intestinal phase causes the various gastrointestinal associated symptoms of nausea, vomiting, diarrhea, rheumatism, backaches, stomach aches, headaches, fever and abdominal pain, while the invasion of skeletal and cardiac muscle by the new larvae results in the various other symptoms associated with Trichinosis. From there, the worms work themselves into the spinal cord and travel the spinal cord toward the brain, at which time there is no possible cure.

What I want for you to overstand is that this unclean animal carry parasites that live in your brain and when you consume this animal it alters your behavior. You are not in your normal state of mind because of the parasites that control you. It is to my overstanding that pork eaters are violent and irrational individuals who are very difficult to reason with. Many foods that we eat and products that we use contain pork or pork byproducts so become familiar with reading the labels.

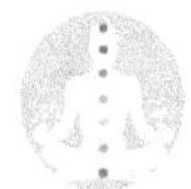

Foods and everyday products that contain pork that you may not have know about

We have to be careful and learn to read the labels of everything that we consume. I say this with the purpose of educating you on how most companies will use scientific terms to hide the names of the item used. I have the names listed.

- Gelatin, which is made from animal bones and tendons
- Casein or milk fat
- Lard
- Refined cane sugar, which may be processed with charred bone fragments
- Carmine, which is used in some artificial color and confectioner's glaze, and is made from beetles
- E 904, E 120, 901, 904, 542, all of which are derived from animals

Gelatine is used in a variety of ways, not just by the food industries. Gelatin comes from a pig source made from bones, cartilage, tendons, and skin of the pig. it can be used as a gelling agent, thickener, film former, adhesive agent, stabilizer, or whipping agent.

When you google Casein you find that Casein protein is a protein found in milk that gives milk its white color. Cow's milk consists of around 80% casein protein. In addition to milk, casein protein is found in yogurt, cheese, and infant formulas, as well as in a variety of dietary supplements. Do not confuse casein protein with casein peptides.

Lard is a semi-solid white fat product obtained by rendering the fatty tissue of a pig. Like butter or shortening, lard is a cooking fat that can be used for baking, sauteing, grilling, or

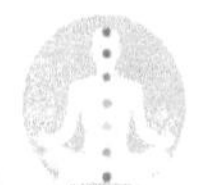

frying. Many big name restaurants use this method for cooking their food.

Refined Sugar are typically used to add flavor to foods but can also act as a preservative in jams and jellies or help foods like pickles and breads ferment. They're also often used to add bulk to processed foods like soft drinks and ice cream.

Carmine (cochineal beetle) is one of the most used natural dyes because it works well on food giving them a shade that ranges from pink to deep red. It can be used in syrups, sweets, jams, gums, industrial cakes, canned vegetables, ice creams and dairy products, such as strawberry or wild berry yogurt, or in some energy drinks.

Besides, in the meat industry, it is indeed the most popular dye being used for all products in this category such as sausages, chorizos, hams and other products made from poultry and pork.

Common Sources of Gelatin:
1. Gelatin desserts like Jell-O
2. Fruit Snacks and gummy candies
3. Marshmallows
4. Circus Peanuts
5. Candy Corn
6. Frosted Mini Wheats
7. Meats–aspics, head cheese, glazed or canned hams
8. Gravies, sauces
9. Medications and supplements
10. Beer, wine, juices
11. Nerds (contains pork gelatin)
12. Altoids (contains pork gelatin)

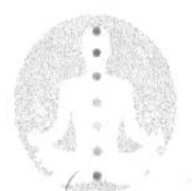

Common Sources of Casein:
- cow's milk
- goat's milk
- Cream
- half and half
- yogurt
- sour cream
- Ice cream
- butter
- cheese
- pudding
- cream-based soups
- sherbet
- custard

Common sources of Refined Sugar
- ice cream.
- candy.
- pastries.
- cookies.
- soda.
- fruit juices.
- canned fruit.
- processed meat.

Common Sources of Carmine
- candies
- ketchup
- soft drinks
- canned cherries
- Ice cream
- Processed meats

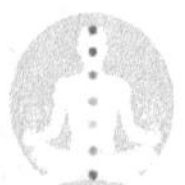

I will list many products that contain pork and do forgive if I leave any out.

Cheese! Many cheeses are made with animal enzymes which are used to thicken milk during the first stages of the cheese making process. Though some cheese brands use cow enzymes, you have to do some deep research to find out which kind of enzymes your cheese brand uses. To be honest most companies that list "enzymes" instead of listing which animal it came from usually means it came from a pig source. Most pizza places buy cheese in bulk to make many pizzas to mass produce them and they want the most cost-effective cheese for business to make money. It will cost them a lot more to buy cheese with vegetarian or microbial enzymes UPDATE: Microbial enzymes are produced by bacteria, fungi, and yeast. Therefore, most will opt for cheese with pig enzymes.

Products like Doritos, Cheetos, Welches grape jelly, Dunkin donuts, crest tooth paste, McDonald's apple pies, and gummy bears contain pig enzymes. Look out for powdered cheese flavoring on chips and store-bought macaroni with cheese which can contain casein, whey, or animal-derived enzymes. SOME Doritos products contain pork.Frito Lay, the makers of Doritos use a pork enzyme called porcine in SOME of their products.

I would be cautious with such products.
If you have any doubts to which products contain pork always call the company and ask them and get more information.

Bread! Pre-made loaves of bread from the grocery store, bagels, breadsticks etc. Most bread that is purchased from the store

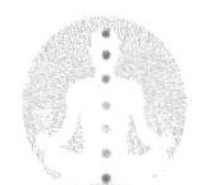

and even bakeries, are made using a dough conditioner called L-cysteine which are certain proteins gathered from the hair and follicles of animals including pigs. Some sources say that L-cysteine contains human hair as well. The regulations for our food is so loose that manufacturers are allowed to manipulate terms and lead people astray.

Fast food grease! Be careful that they do not fry their foods in lard, because lard comes from pork fat. Jiffy corn bread mix is unclean because it contains lard as well. Keratin also known as (PHK) is pig hairs, feathers, hoofs, claws, horns etc.

Mono and diglycerides are food additives used as an emulsifier for commercial foods. They derive it from a fatty acid called E471 produced from vegetable oils, although animal's fats are sometimes used and cannot be completely excluded as being present in the product. This additive is found in breads, ice cream, margarine (I can't believe it's not butter) , some peanut butter, mission tortillas, Nestle cocoa, Country Crock, Blue bonnet, gum, shortening, whipped toppings, marshmallows, and some beverages. Be careful what you pick up and eat and if you are unsure they call the manufacturer to determine if they are using a vegetable or animal fatty acid.

Look out for supplements like fish oil that contains a gelatin capsule that contains the fish inside of it. If it doesn't specify what kind of gelatin they are using like bovine (beef) or vegetable gelatin, it is going to be pig gelatin.

Majority of beer and wines use Isinglass which is a gelatin like substance collected from the bladders of freshwater fish like

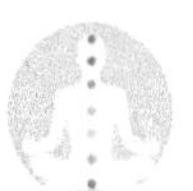

a Sturgeon which is used to clarify the alcohol. Other agents commonly used are egg white albumen, gelatin (pig) and casein. Make sure you look for vegan wine that uses clay or a clean fish to filter the alcohol.

Toothpaste is another product that is made from pig. The fat that is extracted from its bones is incorporated in making many types of toothpastes to give it texture.

Ivory Soap
Animal fats in Ivory are the usually discarded tallow of beef and pork. In addition, animal fats are the main ingredients in Ivory, making up over fifty percent of the product.

Currently US labeling laws do not require manufacturers to cite the source of the gelatin, be it from bovine (cows) or porcine (pork).

- Wine: Gelatin, a product derived from pig body parts, is used in many wine purification processes.

- Baking goods: Cysteine is used in many baking goods such as bread, to create a more extensible dough with improved pan flow. Cysteine is most often synthesised from hair, such as pig bristles.

- Cereal: Many cereals are sugar coated which can also contain gelatin.

- Yogurt: Gelatin is used in many products, especially in the low-calorie variety.

- Fruit Gum: Again gelatin is used in the production of fruit gums.

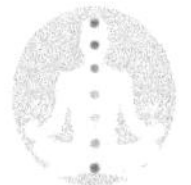

- Chewing Gum: Stearic acid is used in many chewing gums. It is obtained from animal fats, mostly from a pig's stomach.

- Instant soup: Some seasonings in soup contain traces of bacon.

- Cream Cheese: In some products, gelatin is used as a thickener.

- Chips: 'Bacon flavour' is used in some branded products to enhance the flavour.

- Juice: For purification of some juice (especially multivitamin-juice) gelatin is used.

Collagen is the most abundant protein in the body and is a major component of our bones, skin, muscle tendons and cartilage.

People have sought out collagen and gelatin supplements with the hopes of strengthening their hair, nails and improving the elasticity of their skin akin to a fountain of youth.

Alternatives

Luckily there is a balance and it's good to know many companies provide comparable products made with vegetarian agar or carrageenan.

Sour, Gummy, and Hard Candies that are Vegan-Friendly

Below is a list of vegan-friendly candies that you can consume without the worry of accidentally consuming pork gelatin or another animal product:

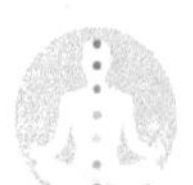

- Airheads
- Some varieties of Jolly Ranchers
- Cracker Jacks
- Smarties
- RJ's Raspberry Soft-Eating Licorice
- Skittles
- Sweet's Fish (Non-GMO)
- Sweet's Lotsa sour candies
- Blow Pops
- Sweet's Lemonade Rings
- Dots
- Sweet's sour worms

Vegan-Friendly Chocolate Candy

Dark chocolate is actually completely plant-based rather than being made with dairy products.

Some of the best vegan candies happen to be chocolate! I have listed some go-to brands to fill your chocolate cravings:

- Crispy Cat Chocolate Bars
- Newman's Own Dark Chocolate Varieties
- Kallari Chocolates
- Alter Eco Dark Chocolate Varieties

Sweets and Gelatin and Alternative Options

Jell-O and Gelatin Dessert Alternatives

J-E-L-L-O....

If you are avoiding pork gelatin there are several options to choose from when making a vegan gelatin-like dessert.

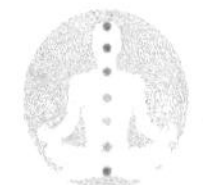

Simply Delish Jel Dessert packages come in a variety of fruit flavors and all are made with carrageenan.

Bakol brand Jel Dessert's are vegan and kosher are also available in a variety of fruit flavors as well as unflavored.

Marshmallow Alternatives

There are several marshmallow companies that offer vegan and vegetarian options.

Yummallo offers several uniquely flavored marshmallows but currently the only gelatin-free option is their vegan option so double check the label before purchasing.

(Dandies is another vegan marshmallow manufacturer that produces regular and mini marshmallows in addition to flavored varieties including maple, pumpkin and peppermint.)

Trader Joe's have numerous vegan and vegetarian offerings has their own line of gelatin free marshmallows!

Lots of options to try for your next smores campfire or rice treat recipes.

Circus Peanuts Alternatives

These fluffy orange marshmallow candies likely fall into the love them or hate them category along with candy corn.

(According to the Spangler Candy company, the most well known manufacturer of circus peanuts, states that the original marshmallow treats were invented in the 1800's and first produced by the Spangler Candy Company on March 12, 1941.)

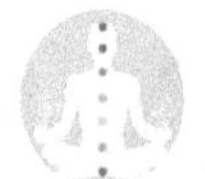

Interestingly enough the iconic orange colored peanut candy is actually banana flavored!

While other flavors including vanilla, lemon and cherry are made, by far the orange version is the most recognized.

Fruit Snacks and Gummy Candy Alternatives
Brands like Annie's make Organic Bunny Fruit Snacks are organic, gluten free and vegan/gelatin free opting to use ingredients like tapioca syrup solids and pectin to provide the gummy consistency gelatin typically provides.

This brand has many flavors like berry, strawberry, raspberry, apple and pink lemonade you're sure to find one you enjoy.

Trader Joes has a Swedish fish alternative called Scandinavian Swimmers Gummy Candy Fish that are gelatin-free and are made with tapioca starch and cornstarch.

Sweet Smarts Sweet Fish are also gelatin-free and lower in sugar using ingredients like allulose and monk fruit to provide chewiness and less sugar than traditional Swedish fish.

Surf Sweets Organic Fruity Bears would be a good one to try in lieu of traditional gummy bears.

Which is with organic fruit juice, plant-based colors, non-GMO, Kosher-Parve, gluten free and no corn syrup

There is still plenty of sugar and no nutritional benefit but a great treat to enjoy while avoiding gelatin.

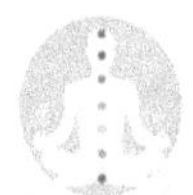

Sweetened Cereal Alternatives

There are fewer good options when looking for an alternative to Kellogg's Frosted Mini Wheats though Kashi cereals may be your closest option.

Kashi's whole wheat biscuits come in four flavor options including berry bountiful, island vanilla, cinnamon harvest and plain autumn wheat.

Meats and Sources of Gelatin

Chances are if you are avoiding pork gelatin, many of the meat products that contain gelatin are also pork products such as canned ham or aspics.

It is always better for you to prepare your own meals at home so you can have more control over the types of ingredients you want to include or avoid.

Gravies and Sauces

While some restaurants and commercially prepared gravies and sauces may contain gelatin, many are thickened with simple cornstarch or other vegetable based thickeners.

Read the labels on your favorite brands to confirm if gelatin of any kind is used.

Medications and Supplements

Obvious forms of gelatin within medications and supplements are found within those that use a soft gel capsule or within the coating or liquids.

Talk to your doctor or pharmacist to determine if alternatives are available for your prescription or supplement.

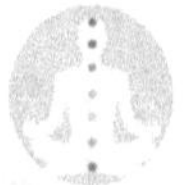

Crimes linked to pork
Man stabbed former colleague in five-year feud over sausage roll

Matthew Evans, 36, barged into a terrified woman's home in Hemel Hampstead and told her he had just stabbed someone moments after the knife attack - and bizarrely asked for a lift away from the scene. Evans stabbed the man in the abdomen five years after accusing the victim of eating his sausage roll

NEWS
FIGHT OVER PORK CHOPS ENDS IN DEATH, POLICE SAY
Chicago Tribune
Aug 12, 1987 at 12:00 am

A South Side man was charged with murder early Tuesday after police said he stabbed a fellow tenant to death after an argument over who would get the larger portion of pork chops during dinner.

The suspect, Mr. Jones, 53, and the victim, Mr. Giles, 27, were having a late dinner Monday night in a house they shared with several other men at 8833 S. Luella Ave., according to Lt. Philip Cline of the Pullman Area violent crimes unit

Mar 7, 2022
Argument over pork chops turns violent; Man arrested for stabbing

An argument over pork chops turned violent after one man's hunger erupted into a full out attack, leaving the victim stabbed and bleeding, and resulting in an arrest.

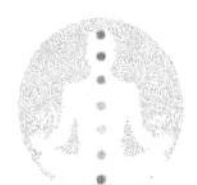

Mr. Bolden, 74, is charged with assault and battery with a deadly weapon after his arrest March 6.

Uncle accused of stabbing nephew over pork chop

Billy Wall accused of stabbing nephew with butcher knife

Updated: 9:12 AM EDT Oct 22, 2014

FELLSMERE, Fla. —
An argument over pork chops turned violent and bloody between relatives Monday night.

Fellsmere police arrested Mr. Wall for stabbing his nephew with a butcher knife two times in the abdomen. The two were apparently arguing over how many pork chops each person would get to eat.

Fight over last rib at barbecue results in victim being stabbed with fork

MUNCIE, Ind. (May 27, 2015) — One woman was hospitalized and another arrested after a fight over the last rib at a backyard barbecue turned violent.

The fight broke out on North Turner Street in Muncie on Sunday night. Officers got a call about a stabbing around 7 p.m., in the midst of a large family barbecue.

According to a police report obtained by the Muncie Star Press, a woman told police she had been stabbed in the eye with a fork by Ms. Davis, a family friend.

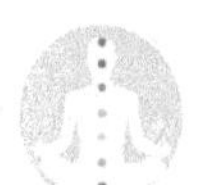

"She was upset that Davis was taking the last rib from the kitchen," an officer said in the report. "(She) then confronted Davis about taking all the food."

During the confrontation, the victim said Davis was using a fork to take meat from a pan when she turned and used the fork to stab her in the eye.

That victim was taken to the hospital for lacerations and a swollen eye and later released.

Davis told officers she was acting in self-defense, after the victim pulled out a knife during the argument

Woman threatens to stab brother with 10-inch butcher knife for eating her BBQ ribs
Published October 1, 2015
FOX 5 Atlanta

Austin Police Department
Austin Police say 61-year-old Ms. Banks tried to stab her brother for eating her barbecue ribs.According to court paperwork, the woman's brother called police, Sunday, September 27th and told them his sister became enraged after finding out someone had eaten her ribs.The bother explained to Banks he didn't know they belonged to her. However, the apology was not enough for Banks and she pushed him. In true brother-sister fashion he pushed her right back; that is when the barbecue debacle got out of control.Officials say, Banks went into the kitchen; grabbed a 10-inch butcher knife; held it over her head; and screamed out she was going to kill her sibling

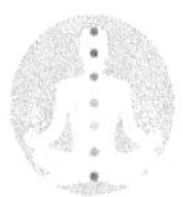

APRIL 10, 2018 10:15 PM
Georgia man fires pistol when wife brings him wrong barbecue ribs, cops say

Mr. Danielly is charged with aggravated assault. Monroe County Jail.

There was an emergency call on a recent Saturday night just west of Rock Branch on the south side of Forsyth.

Word was that someone had been shot at a house on Willis Wilder Drive.

But when Monroe County sheriff's deputies got there, they soon learned that the only thing with a bullet hole in it was a bedroom door.

Now that we have learned a brief history of the pig we must learn to disassociate ourselves from it entirely. Now we have to cleanse and detox ourselves to set forth good health which is true wealth.

Eat But Don't Pig Out
The Right way to eat and heal your body

There are many foods I wish to teach you not to eat, but so many of you cannot avoid eating them.

We must prepare and grow our own food, because this is a highly commercialized world. They genetically modify a lot of food, and some of this food is not good for our stomachs.

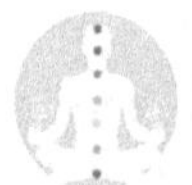

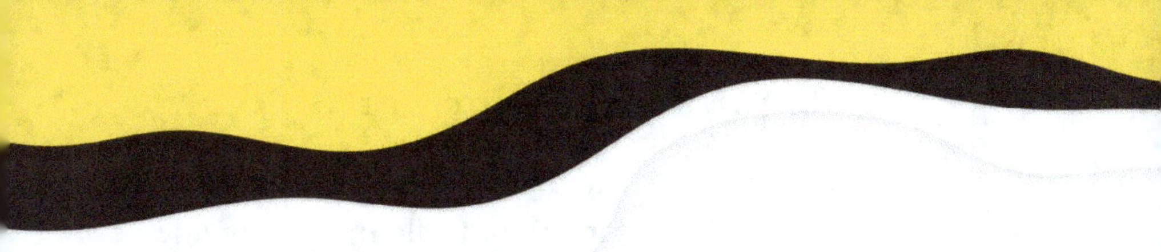

OTHER FOODS THAT WE SHOULD NOT EAT

Bread is a food that we should learn to stay away from because after bread is consumed it still rises.

The rising of bread dough occurs rapidly, and the dough continues to expand in the warm and wet environmetnt of the stomach. This ongoing expansion of material can cause bloat, foreign body obstruction, stomach torsion, hypovolemic shock, and in very severe cases stomach rupture.

All bread will rise again in our stomachs buckling our stomach and intestinal walls. The more it is cooked, the less this will happen.

If you can not break the habit of eating bread then I would suggest eating Rye Bread but it has to be cooked enough times in order for it to be eaten I wouldn't recommend eating this bread if you're someone who is not physically active because your body must be able to break it down. Whole-wheat bread cooked thoroughly is the best bread to eat.

Soy bean flour is very rich, and not good for our stomachs. Our stomachs are too delicate for soy bean flour, therefore, leave those beans alone.

The lima bean is another large bean advertised for you to eat. which will almost burst the lining of the stomach and intestines of an animal 5 times your size.

Milk is also another thing that we should stay away from because it is allowed to have over 750,000 somatic cells (Puss) and 24,000 live bacteria present in it before it violates the food administration guidelines. Also when it says it is pasteurized that's a process that uses radiation to prolong the shelf life of the milk it has sulfur containing amino acids in which throws of the balance of the PH balance of the human body.

Marijuana is not a food but I suggest that men do not smoke this herb but ingest it instead because when you heat it the chemicals properties change. Many states have begun to legalize marijuana which is very detrimental to our health. Legal marijuana that is being grown have pesticides and synthetic estrogen and are magnesium and manganese inhibitors. Mainly men should stay away from marijuana because we cannot produce zinc and zinc and testosterone work together to create semen.

Many foods contain estrogen such as preservatives (sodium benzoate)

Meat is another food that I suggest we we stop eating. Based on the way the human body is constructed we were never

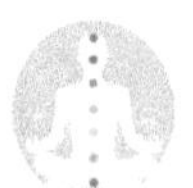

designed to consume and digest meat we don't have elongated Canines **Also known as Cuspids** which are used to tear and rip meat, we would have a short colons and like most carnivorous animals we would sleep 18-20 hours a day. Our body is naturally constructed to how the Most High planned for us to eat.

As the saying goes "you are what you eat" the more you eat animals the more animalistic you become.

It is imperative that we know any and everything that we consume some foods have been genetically engineered or modified which is identified as GMO's.

Genetically Modified Foods
President Obama Signed GMO labeling Bill into law July 29, 2016

WASHINGTON, July 29, 2016 – President Barack Obama quietly signed into law legislation that **prevents states from requiring on-package labeling of genetically modified ingredients**, capping an historic win for farm groups, food companies and the biotech industry.

It is known as the DARK Act. D-A-R-K standing for Denying Americans the Right to Know. It was signed by President Obama without fanfare or major media coverage.

The bill would exempt most current GMO foods from being labeled at all. The FDA further commented that it "may be difficult" for any GMO food to qualify for labeling under the bill. And even for any GE foods that might be covered, the bill

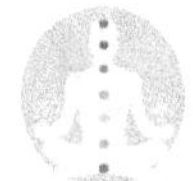

allows for food to be "labeled" through a digital system of QR codes that can only be accessed if the consumer has a smart phone and reliable internet connectivity.

The DARK Act was not subject to any hearings. No expert testimony was taken. Rather, it was the result of backroom dealing between a few senators and industrial food and biotech companies.

The last provision in the bill, added at the 11th hour, allows all organic food to be labeled as "non-GMO" without any testing to see whether it contains any GMO contamination, as can happen with some organic products. So while non-organic companies that want to label "Non-GMO" will have to undergo testing and verification by third-party verifiers like the Non-GMO Project to ensure that they do not have any significant GMO content.

Do you see the games that are being played when it comes to our health? An article goes on to say:

The largest majority of the American People want to have all information about their food available to them when making food purchasing choices. There is substantive debate about the safety of Genetically Modified Foods. While this debate is ignored by much of the mainstream media, the U.S. Legislature, and business leaders, American citizens have a constitutional right to know what is contained in the food they purchase, and how those foods are produced. President Barack Obama has the legal authority to direct the Food and Drug Administration to require labels identifying foods which contain components that have been engineered or altered at

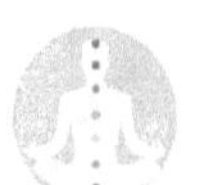

the genetic level. The doctrine of "Substantial Equivalence" that was established by international agreement, and imposed upon the American people by the Administration of George H.W. Bush essentially violates the first amendment rights of American to choice by prohibiting the labeling of products containing components that were produced via means where the science is not only incomplete, but is also disputed. President Barack Obama has the legal authority to, just as the Administration of George H.W. Bush did, determine how a product is labeled by instructing the FDA to require labeling of all Genetically Modified components of foods. This needs to be done immediately. There is no reason that such labeling should not exist, even if it is determined later on that some Genetically Modified components are, in fact, safe. We require that substances on the Generally Recognized As Safe list be included on food labels, and the exemption of GMO components is a clear surrender of the constitutional rights of Americans to special interests that fear that informed people will demand further study of GMO safety.

Foods that Age You

I truly hope that you are still walking with me on this health journey because now I'm about to expose to you all the foods that make you look old. To all my beautiful women I truly hope that you are paying attention to these foods and drinks that I'm about to name.

Black tea
Coffee

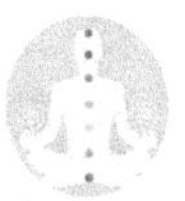

energy drinks (their high caffeine and sodium content can lead to dehydration and dehydration is one of the main factors that contribute to wrinkles and older looking skin)

Milk
Trans fats
Lemonade

Potato chips (Consuming trans fatty acids stimulate interleukin 6 within the body,)

Microwave Dinners (Frozen meals are notoriously high in sodium. Sodium contributes to water retention and an overall 'puffy,' aged appearance)

Baked Goods(Sugar promotes an unhealthy microbiome and it is also pro-inflammatory which can accelerate the aging process)

Hotdogs (Preservatives used in processed meats may create free radicals within the body. "Free radicals lead to oxidation of your cells and DNA, and they can cause enough damage to lead to cancer or other health conditions.

Bacon(Contains nitrates, a preservative necessary in cured meats.

Sugar (Sugar causes inflammation, which is a major inhibitor to having clear, beautiful skin)

High Glycemic Index Carbs (Foods such as bagels, oatmeal, pretzels, pasta, and cereal, have been proven to accelerate the

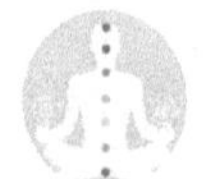

skin's aging process and cause problems with the skin, causing acne and rosacea," Even 'healthy' cereals with whole grains, which are lower in glycemic index, can be stocked full of wrinkle-inducing glucose.

Alcohol (causes free radicals. Alcohol also robs the body of vitamin A, an antioxidant that's essential for cell renewal and turnover)

High Sodium foods(Foods that are high in sodium cause you to retain water and feel bloated. The water retention can make the skin look puffy and tired)

Pepperoni Pizza
The nitrates and other compounds in processed meats, such as pepperoni, are known to be pro-inflammatory. Inflammation causes aging from inside out.

Deep Fried French Fries (When we deep fry foods, we expose the oil and fat to extremely high temperatures and when this happens free radicals are formed)

Fried Fast Food(Restaurants typically use corn oil which is one of the unhealthiest oils and it releases free radicals in the body. Free radical damage or oxidative stress has numerous effects on health and well-being, including heart disease and wrinkles

Agave (this sweet syrup is packed with fructose. Once the liver meets fructose, it not only turns it into fat but also breaks down collagen, making fine lines more noticeable)

Candy(affects dental health and makes you appear to be older)

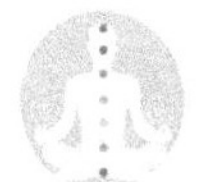

Charred Meat (is very inflammatory to the body,Inflammation may actually break down collagen levels in the skin leading to an aged appearance)

High Fructose Corn Syrup (high fructose corn syrup is believed to be the worst kind for your skin and health it can damage your skin's collagen and elastin, making you look wrinkled with skin that is no longer firm

Canned Soups (high in sodium)

Soda (inflammation-causing sugar is considered to be erosive and is bad for your teeth)

We must learn to eat one meal a day and let it be without pork and many of the ailments that you suffering from and getting medically treated for will disappear.

If you are a diabetic it would be wise to eat one meal a day and lay off starch and sugar because they are only making you sick and in a week your urine will be negative of sugar and acid negative.

I will say that ignorance is suffering with a disease when it can easily be cured. You must stop eating that which is causing your trouble.

I CAN ONLY HELP YOU IF YOU'RE WILLING TO HELP YOURSELF

After I look at the current day conditions of my people it is safe to say that we have been attacked with the heavily commercialized food which is mainly pork and we must learn to live without it.

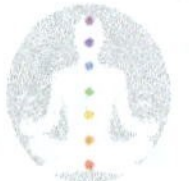

I must say that we have been bred through our genes to love pork and to many that may seem far fetched but scientists have confirmed that emotions good or bad, happy or sad can be passed down through the genes. We must learn to detox ourselves and get rid of all of these toxins and poisons that enter our bodies by way of food consumption.

What I now overstand is that my people's condition is so severe concerning this poisonous swine that they may have to undergo therapy because this is a psychological condition for many of us.

Brief History of Dr. Sebi

Dr. Sebi who's real name was Alfredo Bowman was a herbalist healer who practiced in Honduras and the United States.

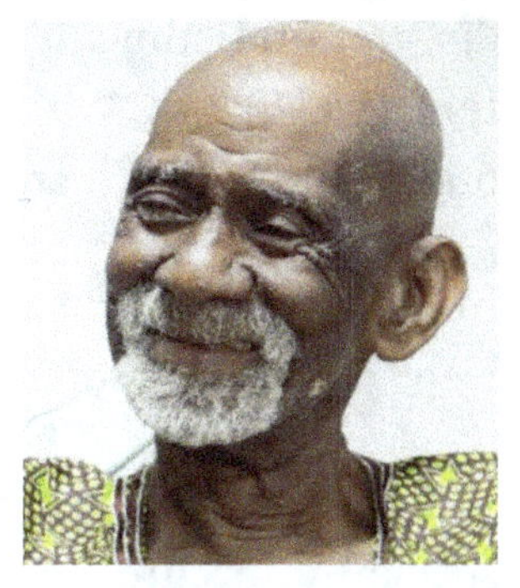

Dr. Sebi First Appeared in the 1980's as a Herbalist, Naturalist, Health Activist

Alfredo Bowman was born in 1933 in Ilanga village in Spanish Honduras. He never had any formal schooling but learned about herbal healing and related traditional practices from his grandmother.

Sebi was diagnosed by a Mexican herbalist named Alfredo Cortez with asthma, diabetes, impotency, and visual impairment. Cortez gave Sebi a death sentence.

After that, Sebi started to experiment on himself with different herbs and fasting methods.

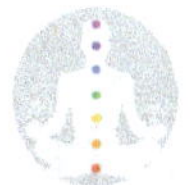

Not only did he heal himself but also started treating people around him.

Dr. Sebi food therapy was based on an alkaline plant-based diet and lots of natural supplements.

Dr. Sebi's second wife gave him the name Sebi and locals started calling him Doctor after they saw him heal illnesses. Sebi had 4 wives and allegedly 20 children from his many romantic relationships.

Dr. Sebi has been CURING (not treating) people suffering from diseases and ailments such as AIDS, DIABETES, PROSTATE INFLAMATION, SICKLE CELL, BLINDNESS among many others, Using only natural Herbs and Minerals from the Earth.

In 1985 Dr. Sebi placed an ad in The Amsterdam News, The New York Post, and The Village, the ad read…..

"Aids has been cured by the Usha Research Institute, and we specialize in cures for Sickle Cell, Lupus, Blindness, Herpes, Cancer and others."

The ad ran for 2 years before he was attacked by the Attorney General of New York. Dr. Sebi was told to remove the ad, when he refused within days he was served with a arrest warrant. According to Dr. Sebi the Attorney General bragged that he was going to "put Dr. Sebi under the jail!" The charges read to the jury was as follows..

Mr. Alfred Bowman aka Dr. Sebi, you are hereby charged with practicing medicine without a license, selling products not approved by the FDA (Federal Drug Administration) and

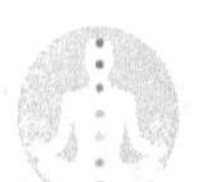

claiming to cure Aids, and other diseases which is a fraudulent claim."

Dr Sebi was told to bring 1 person for each of the diseases he claimed to court with proof from a reputable doctor that the individual had the disease, then proof from another reputable doctor that the person was cured. Instead of bringing 1 for each disease, approx 70 people filled the court all with proof! The judge shook his head according to Dr. Sebi and said I did not ask for all of this. To make a long story short, the judge after seeing the proof and speaking with Dr. Sebi turned to the states attorney and asked, "Did you investigate the man?" She said, "No" The judge then said,

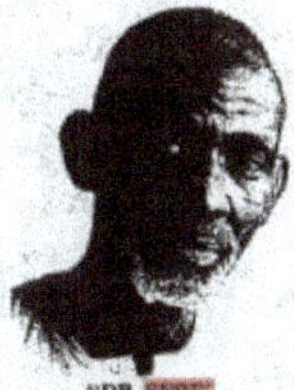

Herbalist found not guilty in 'fake' healing case
HAROLD L JAMISON
New York Amsterdam News (1962-1993); Oct 1, 1988;
ProQuest Historical Newspapers New York Amsterdam News: 1922-1993
pg. 5

Herbalist found not guilty in 'fake' healing case

By HAROLD L. JAMISON

In a historical decision in Brooklyn Supreme Court Monday, a jury of six men and six women found Alfredo Bowman not guilty on two counts of practicing medicine without a license.

Bowman, affectionately known as Dr. Sebi, director of USHA Herbal Research Institute, 616 Pacific St., Brooklyn, was arrested Feb. 10, 1987, by Attorney General Robert Abrams' office because ads placed in the Village Voice and the Amsterdam News, claimed a cure for AIDS.

Simeon Greenaway, Sebi's attorney stated this was the first case of its kind in Brooklyn Supreme Court.

"What was significant about the verdict," Greenaway stated, "is the fact that USHA's African Bio-Mineral Balance will now be recognized throughout the world."

Sebi described the African Bio-Mineral Balance "as a dietary program that is consistent with the African genetic structure."

The dietary program consists of natural herbal compounds, fresh fruits, vegetables and juices.

According to Sebi's testimony, "the compounds change the environment of the body through intra-cellular cleansing and replenish the cells by causing cell proliferation, wherein new cells push out the old cells."

This process enables the body to heal itself.

Greenaway described USHA's concept of natural healing as one "on a collision course with the medical establishment."

Objections to the views being expressed by Sebi prompted the attorney general to wage a "fear and smear" campaign to discredit the reputation of Sebi and the USHA Institute, according to Greenaway.

Abrams proceeded with the case on the "erroneous assumption" that the compounds being marketed were medicinal. However, no attempt was made to ascertain the contents of the herbal compounds before or after the arrest.

During the trial Assistant General Barclay revealed that two undercover agents were sent to the institute on two separate occasions in an attempt "to entrap Sebi into making medical diagnoses." After being briefed by a medical doctor as to the symptoms of a urinary infection and herpes, the undercover agents Gail Malis and Michael Colon were wired with a small tape recorder. The tape recording, submitted into evidence by Barclay, failed to convince the jury that Sebi did in fact make a medical diagnosis. One agent's testimony, under cross examination by Greenaway, clearly stated that he did not receive the response from Sebi that would constitute a medical diagnosis.

A questionnaire used by Sebi to ascertain the health of clients was submitted in evidence by the prosecution to support its contentions that Sebi and the institute were practicing medicine. However, this was dispelled by testimony of Marjorie Thorne-Puckorin, a former USHA employee who testified that individuals were required to fill out the questionnaires to enable the institute to monitor clients health conditions, diet and collect data for research purposes.

Harry Dickson, Roger Marshall, Naimah Fuller, Zadia Ife and Karen Selby, witnesses for the defense, unequivocally testified to their improved health as a result of USHA's dietary program.

"DR. SEBI"

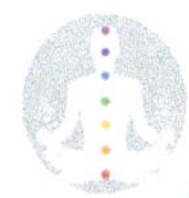

"well, the answer he just gave me, he cures AIDS. You all are in trouble." Dr. Sebi was then found NOT GUILTY on all charges by the state of New York and the supreme court because he was indeed curing people of the various diseases, including AIDS. Dr. Sebi had cured 5 AIDS patients before he put the Ad in the papers. The media asked Dr. Sebi, where are all the so called black leaders??? This is a historical moment! A African American that is curing AIDS in America! Yet none of them have come out to celebrate your victory and make the big announcement.

Disease is a multi billion dollar industry, there's money to be made in sickness. It would not be wise for big pharmaceutical companies to publicly announce that most untreatable diseases are being cured. Do you know how much money sickel cell centers collect each year?!! Cancer Research Centers?? Diabete Centers?? and the list goes on! The prescription companies pay the television shows salary.

Dr. Sebi Cured By Fasting-
Sick and angry to the point of wanting to kill his wife, Dr. Sebi suffered from obesity, impotence, diabetes, asthma and suicidal tendencies. His frustration with impotency caused him to express his illnesses with his associates in hopes that someone could help. He sought remedies from African herbalists to the Chinese, alternative and holistic solutions; oh he tried everything. Eventually a friend of his by the name "Ronald Evans" called him on the phone and told him that he knew a Mexican that could help him. After Dr. Sebi and some of his street partners divided a large sum of money, he bought a car and was soon on his way to Cuernavaca, Mexico to see a

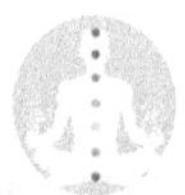

94-year old man by the name of "Alfredo Cortez" who had two wives.

He begins his journey teaching how lactic, carbonic and uric acid are responsible for the amount of deterioration that occurs in the body. These three acids cause what they call uncontrolled mitosis. Starch is carbonic acid.

Dr Sebi has stated that fasting will heal every part of you that you need to be healed.

LISA "LEFT EYE" LOPES
Dr Sebi reports how Lisa Lopes came to him with severe eye twitching, smoking addiction and herpes (of which she did not inform him of until she 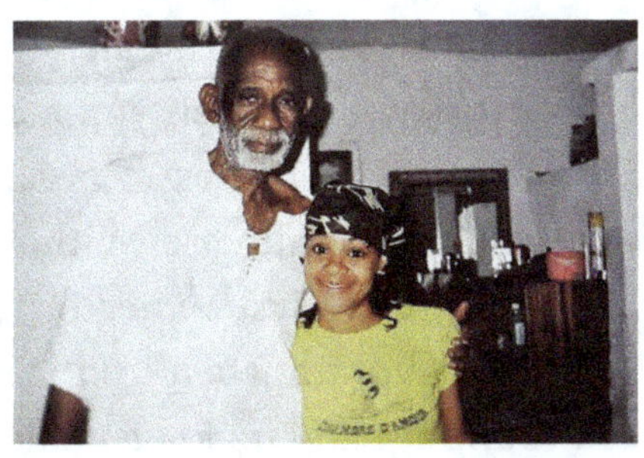 was cured). Dr. Sebi recommended that she fast for 40 days and 40 nights. She drunk a mixture of juiced kale and bromide tea on her fast. Once Lisa was cured of all her illnesses she began promoting Dr. Sebi by holding lectures and organizing trips to Usha Village in Honduras for family and friends.

The task where healing must be accomplished is found in the pH balance in the body's blood. Immunology reveals that getting sick, acquiring diseases and bad microbes are due to a deficiency in the body which affects the immune system. If the pH of the body is acidic, then it will strip the body of it's mineral nutrients and deprived the body's ability to have a strong immune system.

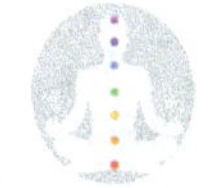

IRON

Dr. Sebi has made some very significant statements in reference to plant-based iron. It is impossible for you to get sick if your iron level is up to par. If you have a disease, no matter what kind of disease it is, you are anemic. Iron is the mineral that conveys oxygen to the brain. Iron should have carbon, hydrogen and oxygen. (the CHO chain). Iron is the spark plug of the human body. When you are deficient in iron, you are susceptible to a whole bunch of diseases. Iron fires the body up and is the only mineral on the planet that is magnetic. Being that iron is magnetic it has a tendency to pull other minerals to it. It pulls magnesium, zinc, gold, calcium, phosphorous, etc. It would be safe to say that when you take large doses of iron that you are taking all the other minerals. The lack of iron causes 40 manifestations of disease. Without iron, the body looses energy and the immune system begins to give way. There is no oxygen going to the brain when iron is low. Without iron, we wrinkle at a young age and no longer able to walk straight. The Burdock plant is rich in iron. The body naturally consumes or uses the amount of 3 table spoons of iron a day. Dr. Sebi recommends 2 table spoons 3 times a day.

Dr. Sebi Used Iron to get rid of Sickle cell anemia.

SICKLE CELL ANEMIA

It is the deprivation of iron fluorine. Sickle Cell Anemia is when the blood plasma has broken down by mucous into a sickle. Mucous sinks into the plasma, into the cell itself, breaks and disunites the cell. Removing the mucous the cell unites again. To maintain that level, you have to feed the patient large doses of iron phosphate. Not ferrous oxide.

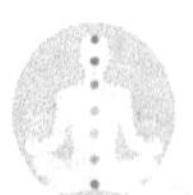

FOOD WITH HIGH IRON CONTENT
Sarsasparilla – Highest content of iron.
Sarsil Berry – Berry from the plant of the sarsasparilla.
Guaco – It's high in iron and strengthens the immune system. Has potassium phosphate.
Conconsa – An African plant. Has the highest concentration of potassium phosphate.
Lily of the Valley – Rich in iron fluorine and Potassium phosphate.
Purslane – Rich in iron.
Kale – Rich in iron.
Dandelion – Rich in iron.
Lams Quarters – Rich in iron.
Burdock – Rich in iron.
Blue Vervain – Rich in iron.
Yellow Dock – Rich in iron.
Chickweed – Rich in iron
Anamu – Rich in iron
Amaranth-Rich in iron

Sebi developed a treatment called the "African Bio-Electric Cell Food Therapy", and claimed that it could cure a wide range of diseases including AIDS and cancer.

He also started marketing and selling herbal products in the Honduras and USA.

In 1988 Dr. Sebi was accused and sent to trial for practicing medicine without a license. Dr Sebi showed up to court barefoot and won the lawsuit, after proving he was not practicing allopathic western medicine. More than 70 people testified to being relieved of their diagnosis after following Dr. Sebi's diet.

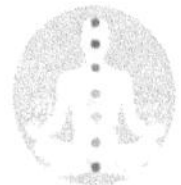

Dr. Sebi created USHA Healing village or USHA Research Institute in Honduras, where hundreds of people have traveled to receive treatment for their ailments.

A second lawsuit in 1993 ordered Alfredo to cease claims that his products can treat serious diseases.

Although Sebi's alkaline diet was not backed up by any mainstream scientific evidence, many clients of Sebi claimed they managed to lose weight, detox their body and even heal chronic disease by sticking with Dr. Sebi's alkaline diet.

Evidently, people increased their health conditions and experienced weight loss by following a clean plan based diet, as opposed to the western diet which is full of processed foods, high in sugar and fatty acids.

Dr. Sebi's healing process was done from the outside-in. By combining a balanced diet comprised of unprocessed plant-based foods, lots of water, and some supplements, Sebi claimed to cleanse the body of excess mucus. Sebi claimed that the excess mucus in the body causes most of the modern diseases that people battle with.

Besides the physical healing, Dr. Sebi was a strong supporter of self-love and emotional independence. Dr. Sebi preached that you must have a healthy mind in order to live in a healthy body.

Amongst his many clients, numerous celebrities were among his patients, including Michael Jackson, Lisa 'Left Eye' Lopes, Erykah Badu, Eddie Murphy, and John Travolta.

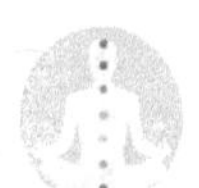

The last case that was brought against Dr. Sebi was on 28 May 2016, Dr. Sebi and his associate were arrested on charges of money laundering. Sebi was kept in a Honduran prison where he got critically ill of pneumonia. Dr. Sebi died on 6 August 2016, on the way to the hospital.

Sebi's arrest and death are questioned by some people that believe that his teachings and treatments were considered a threat by the medical establishment and the pharmaceutical industry.

To this day, Sebi receives a lot of criticism from the science community. His name is also tied to a few conspiracy theories that involve Lisa Left-Eye Lopez or Nipsey Hussle.

Sebi's recipes are very popular amongst the vegan and vegetarian communities. His nutritional guides for weight management and a balanced diet are marketed as diet e-books or courses by nutritionists and health activists.

Dr. Sebi doesn't recommend eating any foods not on the Dr. Sebi food list.

As I stated earlier, the Dr Sebi food list is very specific and excludes many whole-food plant-based foods.

Dr. Sebi Food List

Note: Dr. Sebi has (added) and (removed) items for the food list and is noted so you will have to decide whether you want to still use them.

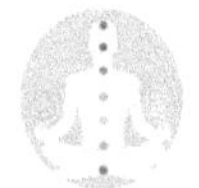

Vegetables

Amaranth greens – same as Callaloo, a variety of Spinach Wild
Arugula (added)

Avocado
Asparagus – (removed)
Bell Peppers
Chayote (Mexican Squash)
Cucumber
Dandelion greens
Garbanzo beans (chick peas)
Green Banana – (removed)
Izote – cactus flower/ cactus leaf- grows naturally in California
Jicama – (removed)
Kale
Lettuce (all, except Iceberg)
Mushrooms (all, except Shitake)
Mustard greens (removed)
Nopales – Mexican Cactus
Okra (added back after being removed)
Olives (and olive oil)
Onions
Parsley (removed)
Purslane (Verdolaga) – (added)
Poke salad -greens (removed)
Sea Vegetables (wakame/dulse/arame/hijiki/nori)
Squash
Spinach – (removed)
String beans – (removed)
Tomato – cherry and plum only
Tomatillo

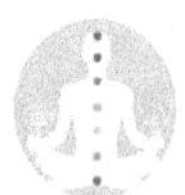

Turnip greens
Watercress – (added)
Zucchini

Fruit
(No canned fruits or Seedless fruits)

Apples
Bananas – the smallest one or the Burro/mid-size (original banana) Berries – all varieties- Elderberries in any form – no cranberries Cantaloupe
Cherries
Currants
Dates
Figs
Grapes -seeded
Limes (key limes preferred with seeds)
Mango
Melons -seeded
Orange (Seville or sour preferred, difficult to find)
Papayas
Peaches
Pears
Plums
Prickly Pear (Cactus Fruit) – (added)
Prunes
Raisins -seeded
Soft Jelly Coconuts (and coconut oil)
Soursops – (Latin or West Indian markets)
Sugar apples (chermoya) – (removed)
Tamarind – (added)

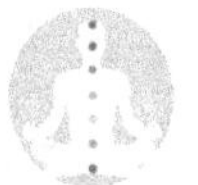

Nuts & Seeds
(Includes nut & seed butters)

Brazil Nuts – (added)
Hemp Seed (added)
Hazelnuts – (removed)
Pine Nuts – (removed)
Raw Almonds and Almond butter- (removed) Raw Sesame Seeds
Raw Sesame "Tahini" Butter Walnuts

Oils
(New Section added by Dr. Sebi) Minimize the use of oils.

Olive Oil (Do not cook)
Coconut Oil (Do not cook)
Grapeseed Oil (added)
Sesame Oil (added)
Hempseed Oil (added) Avocado Oil (added)

Spices – Seasonings
Achiote
Allspice (removed)
Basil
Bay leaf
Cayenne/African Bird Pepper
Cilantro (removed)
Cloves
Coriander (removed)
Cumin (removed)
Dill

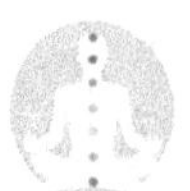

Habanero (added)
Marjoram (removed)
Onion Powder
Oregano
Parsley (removed)
Powdered Granulated Seaweed (Kelp/Dulce/Nori – has "sea taste") Pure Sea Salt
Sage
Savory (added)
Sweet Basil (added)
Tarragon
Thyme

Sugars

100% Pure Agave Syrup – (from cactus)
Date "Sugar – (from dried dates)
100% Pure Maple Syrup – Grade B recommended – (removed)
Maple "Sugar" (from dried maple syrup) – (removed)

Alkaline Grains

Amaranth
Black Rice – (removed)
Fonio – (added) Kamut
Quinoa
Rye
Spelt
Tef
Wild Rice

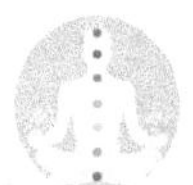

Nutritional Guide | All Natural Herbal Teas
Alvaca (removed)
Anise (removed)
Burdock (added)
Chamomile Elderberry Fennel
Ginger
Lemon grass (removed)
Red Raspberries

It is important to eat living foods that give you energy because as you heard "You Are What You Eat" any time we eat we should feel energized.

The Importance of Healthy Natural Sugars

Most people believe that our bodies can't break down the sugar that's in fruit. There are 3 main bases of sugar which are Galactose Fructose and Glucose

Galactose - Is produced naturally in women's breast milk
Fructose- is naturally occurring in fruit
Glucose- is naturally occurring in vegetables
Diabetes 1&2 can be cured by way of fructose

When you eat fructose it bypasses the pancreas (the pancreas have **islet cells (islets of Langerhans)**that create and release important hormones directly into the bloodstream. You have alpha cells that produce glycogen and you have beta cells that produce insulin then you have the delta cells that produce somatostatin (A mixture of a growth pituitary hormone that is mixed with glycogen.

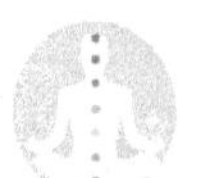

Fructose, galactose and glucose are all monosaccharides. These monosaccharides combine in various pairs to form the three disaccharides that are most important in human nutrition: lactose, maltose and sucrose. The monosaccharide glucose is the common thread in each of these disaccharides.

When fruit or vegetables are cooked their chemical properties change from fructose to dextrose or sucrose (polysaccharides)

Monosaccharides are natural sugars from fruit and vegetables while polysaccharides are created in labs

Someone who is suffering from diabetes normally have a parasite in their pancreas and you discover that is has mucus and the adrenal glands are down and the adrenal are in charge of the autonomic nervous system such as digestion which is controlled by the parasympathetic nervous system. Your body is supposed to automatically be able to convert the glucose into simple insulin for the pancreas. In other words the pancreas yielding insulin is a nervous system issue because the adrenals are not functioning properly because of the wrong foods that we are consuming which in hand is not opening up our lymphatic system allowing our kidney to filter all of the toxins out of our bodies.

When it comes to digestion there are two different types which is pancreas digestive enzymes that break down the glucose the pancreas yields the Amylase to bring glucose to the cell so that your body has energy. Fructose bypasses the pancreas and goes to the liver which causes cellular infusion where the sugar infuses itself to the cell without use of the pancreas.

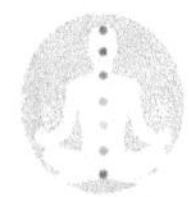

Proper hydration comes with consumption of fruit so fruits are eaten for their macronutrients and water (H302)

Good Sources of (H302):
Berries (oygenators, has antioxidants, have bio photons)
Melons
Coconuts
Cucumber
Mango

When it comes to the type of nutrients our bodies need nature has color coded the fruit of the same color to have the same nutritional properties.

Nutrients in Red Fruits and Vegetables
Lycopene, ellagic acid, Quercetin, and Hesperidin, to name a few.

These nutrients reduce the risk of prostate cancer, lower blood pressure, reduce tumor growth and LDL cholesterol levels, scavenge harmful free-radicals, and support join tissue in arthritis cases.

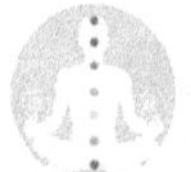

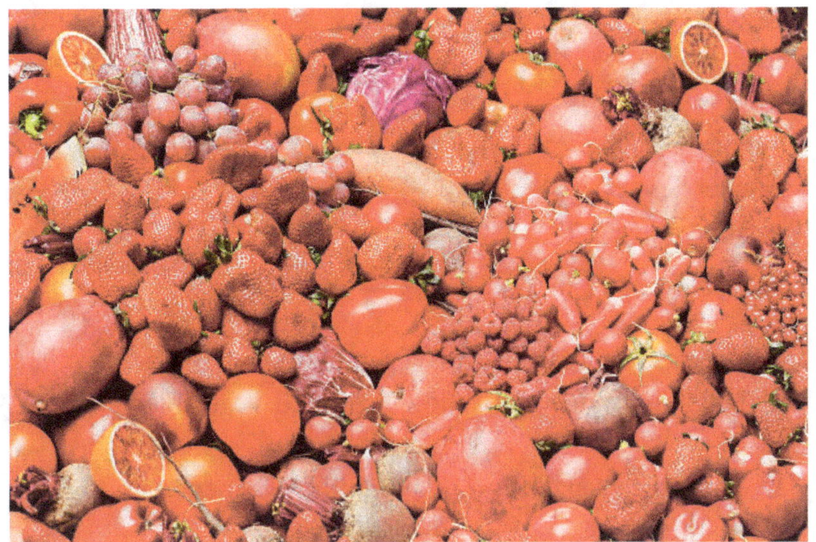

Types of Red Fruits and Vegetables

Beets
Blood oranges
Cherries
Cranberries
Guava
Papaya
Pink grapefruit
Pink/Red grapefruit
Pomegranates
Radicchio
Radishes
Raspberries
Red apples
Red bell peppers
Red chili peppers
Red grapes
Red onions

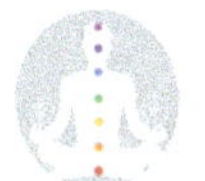

Red pears
Red peppers
Red potatoes
Rhubarb
Strawberries
Tomatoes
Watermelon

Orange and Yellow Fruit and Vegetables
Nutrients in Orange and Yellow Fruit and Vegetables

Beta-carotene, zeaxanthin, flavonoids, lycopene, potassium, and vitamin C.

These nutrients reduce age-related macula degeneration and the risk of prostate cancer, lower LDL cholesterol and blood pressure, promote collagen formation and healthy joints, fight harmful free radicals, encourage alkaline balance, and work with magnesium and calcium to build healthy bones.

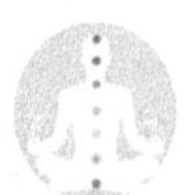

Types of Yellow and Orange Fruits and Vegetables

Apricots
Butternut squash
Cantaloupe
Cape Gooseberries
Carrots
Golden kiwifruit
Grapefruit
Lemon
Mangoes
Nectarines
Oranges
Papayas
Peaches
Persimmons
Pineapples
Pumpkin
Rutabagas
Sweet corn
Sweet potatoes
Tangerines
Yellow apples
Yellow beets
Yellow figs
Yellow pears
Yellow peppers
Yellow potatoes
Yellow summer squash
Yellow tomatoes
Yellow watermelon
Yellow winter squash

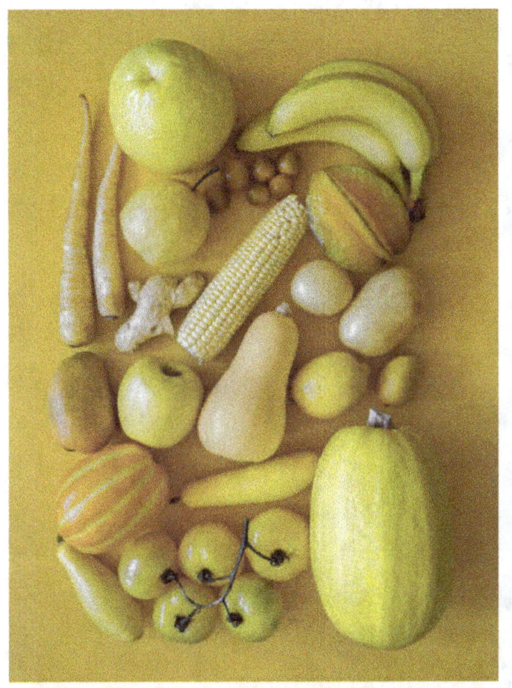

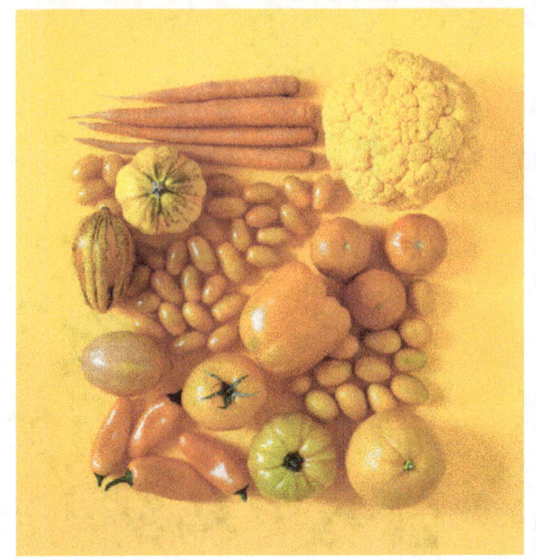

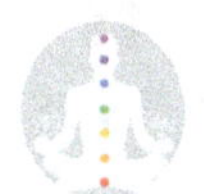

Green Vegetables and Fruit

Nutrients in Green Vegetables and Fruit
Chlorophyll, fiber, lutein, zeaxanthin, calcium, folate, vitamin C, iron, calcium, and Beta-carotene.

The nutrients found in these vegetables reduce cancer risks, lower blood pressure and LDL cholesterol levels, normalize digestion time, support retinal health and vision, fight harmful free-radicals, and boost immune system activity.

Types of Green Fruits and Vegetables
Artichokes
Arugula
Asparagus
Avocados
Broccoflower
Broccoli
Broccoli rabe
Brussel sprouts

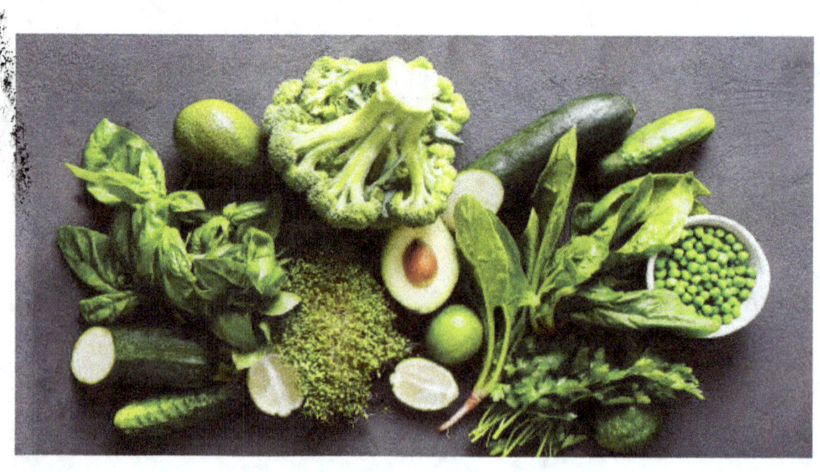

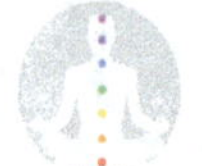

Celery
Chayote squash
Chinese cabbage
Cucumbers
Endive
Green apples
Green beans
Green cabbage
Green grapes
Green onion
Green pears
Green peppers
Honeydew
Kiwifruit
Leafy greens
Leeks
Lettuce
Limes
Okra
Peas
Snow Peas
Spinach
Sugar snap peas
Watercress
Zucchini

Blue and Purple Fruits and Vegetables

Nutrients in Blue and Purple Fruits and Vegetables

Lutein, zeaxanthin, resveratrol, vitamin C, fiber, flavonoids, ellagic acid, and quercetin.

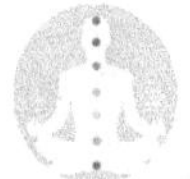

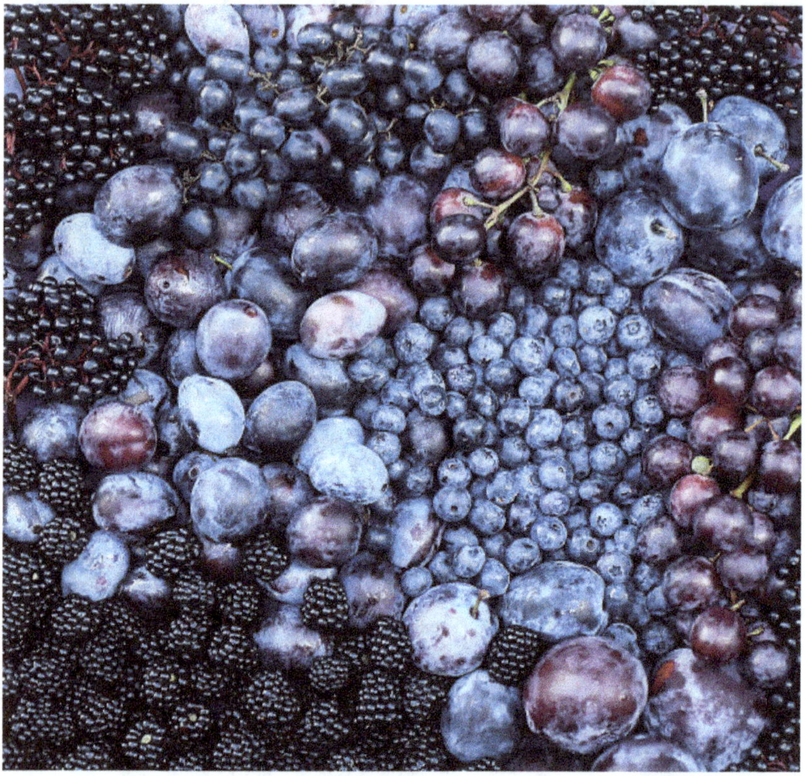

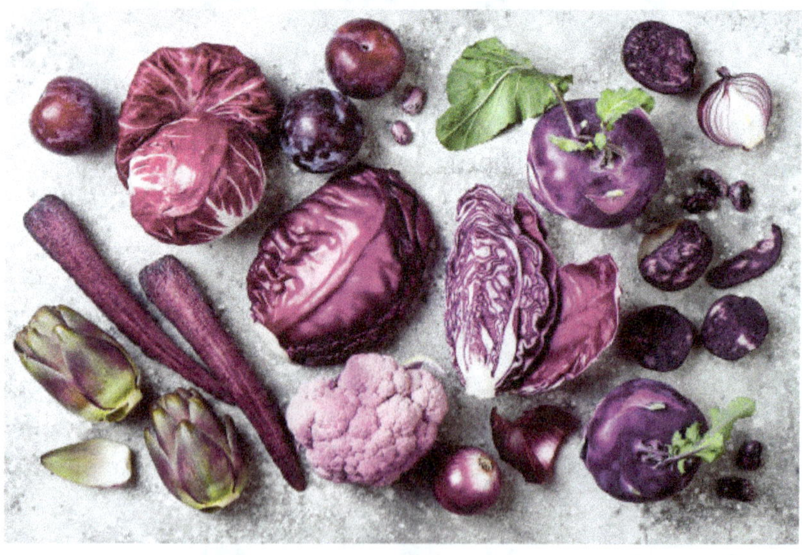

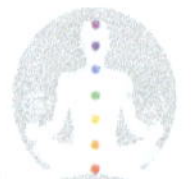

Similar to the previous nutrients, these nutrients support retinal health, lower LDL cholesterol, boost immune system activity, support healthy digestion, improve calcium and other mineral absorption, fight inflammation, reduce tumor growth, act as an anticarcinogens in the digestive tract, and limit the activity of cancer cells.

Types of Blue and Purple Fruits and Vegetables
Black currants
Black salsify
Blackberries
Blueberries
Dried plums
Eggplant
Elderberries
Grapes
Plums
Pomegranates
Prunes
Purple Belgian endive
Purple Potatoes
Purple asparagus
Purple cabbage
Purple carrots
Purple figs
Purple grapes
Purple peppers
Raisins

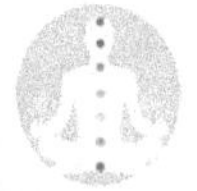

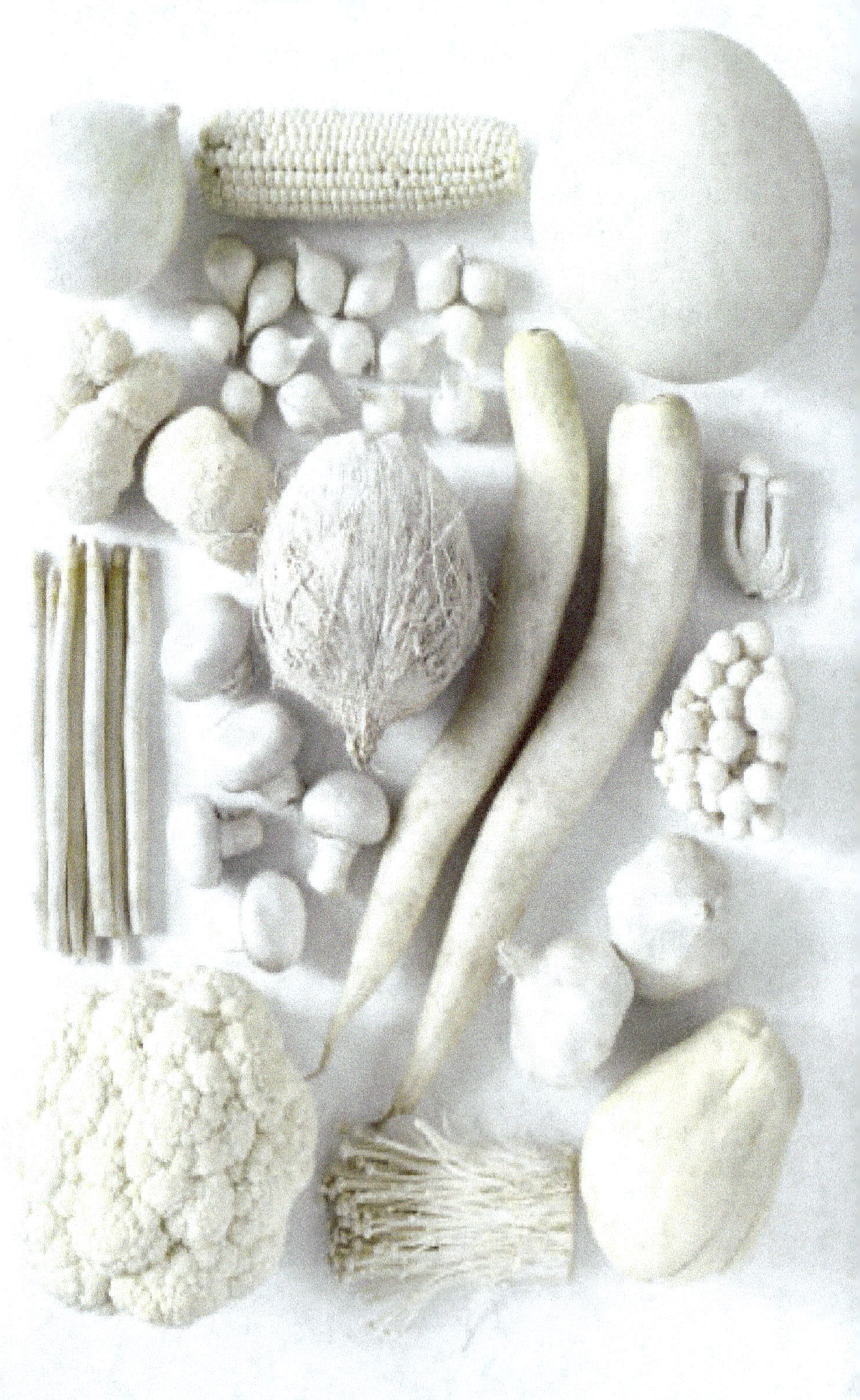

White Colored Fruits and Vegetables
Nutrients in White fruits and Vegetables

Beta-glucans, EGCG, SDG, and lignans that provide powerful immune boosting activity. These nutrients also activate natural killer B and T cells, reduce the risk of colon, breast, and prostate cancers, and balance hormone levels, reducing the risk of hormone-related cancers.

Types of White Fruits and Vegetables
Bananas
Brown pears
Cauliflower
Dates
Garlic
Ginger
Jerusalem artickoke
Jicama
Kohlrabi
Mushrooms
Onions
Parsnips
Potatoes
Shallots
Turnips
White Corn
White nectarines
White peaches

I CAN ONLY HELP YOU IF YOU'RE WILLING TO HELP YOURSELF

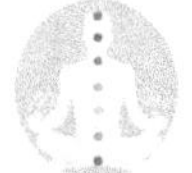

Learning to detox to rid the body of impurities

It is very imperative that we detox all of these harmful things that we consume out of our system so that we can heal ourselves.

Also called detoxification, detox is the process of clearing the toxins and impurities from your body.

The Master Teacher Dr. Malachi Z. York El known as Paa Nabab Yaanuwn said that the Anunnaqi gave us watermelon to cleanse our system because we were being fed to much pork. Watermelon is one of the main foods that has the ability to cleanse your body from all the toxic and impure foods that we eat from day to day.

I will list a few foods that are good for the detoxification of the body especially the main organs. Please be aware that I will not name every food that is good for detoxification but for the ones that I do name should be easily accessible.

FOODS THAT HAVE DETOXIFICATION EFFECTS

Asparagus

Asparagus contains glutathione, a well-known antioxidant that promotes detoxification. It is also a good source of fiber, folate, iron, and vitamins A, C, E, and K, as well as being beneficial to those with high blood pressure. Asparagus is also known to help the kidney and bladder cleanse itself.

Broccoli

Broccoli contains sulforaphane, which is great for fighting off infectious cells in our bodies. Eating broccoli also helps your

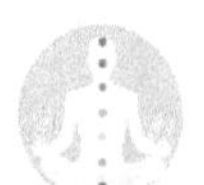

body fight off cancer-inducing chemicals, and boosts the liver's ability to clear bad chemicals from our bodies.

Grapefruit

Grapefruit is loaded with nutrients including vitamins A, C, and B1, as well as pantothenic acid, fiber, potassium, and biotin. Enzymes found in grapefruit may also break down the fat in your body to help promote weight loss. Please note that grapefruit may interact with some medications, so you should speak with your primary care provider before increasing your grapefruit intake.

Avocado

Avocados are loaded with antioxidants that help your body expel harmful toxins. A nutrient-dense food, avocados contain around 20 different vitamins and minerals that help decrease the risk of obesity, diabetes, and heart disease.

(An Avocado is a hybrid food but it has a lot of Omega 3 which is good for the mind. I'm not suggesting that you should or shouldn't eat it but choosing to eat avocados built brain sells.)

Kale

What's the fuss over kale? Packed with amino acids that help keep your mind sharp, kale is also beneficial for managing cholesterol. Kale can also help with managing blood pressure due to its high levels of magnesium and potassium.

Artichokes

Give your liver a break! Artichokes provide a wide variety of nutrients for your blood and liver. Two phytonutrients found

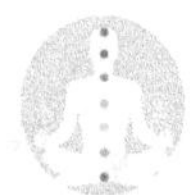

in artichokes help the liver produce bile, which is important in the digestion of fats.

Collard greens

Collard greens are rich in sulfur-containing compounds that support your body's detoxification process. Not only are they high in vitamins K and A, but collard greens may also lower your risk of breast, colon, and lung cancers due to indole-3-carbinol.

Beets

Beets are a high-antioxidant vegetable that are also rich in nutrients. Beets contain betaine, which helps the liver rid itself of toxins, as well as a fiber called pectin that clears toxins that have been removed from the liver.

Spinach

Spinach is low in calories, but packed with nutrients. Spinach contains vitamins A, C, E, and K, as well as thiamin, folate, calcium, iron, and magnesium—the list goes on! Flavonoids in spinach help keep cholesterol from oxidizing in your body by acting as antioxidants.

Lemon

Lemons are a staple of many detox diets, and there is a good reason for this. Firstly, lemons are packed with antioxidant vitamin C, which is great for the skin and for fighting disease-forming free radicals. Furthermore, the citrus fruit has an alkaline effect on the body, meaning that it can help restore the body's pH balance, benefitting the immune system. Try starting your day with hot water and a slice of lemon to help flush out toxins and cleanse your system.

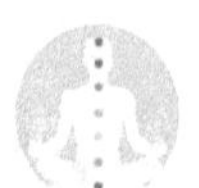

Ginger

If too much fatty food or alcohol has caused problems for your digestive system, it may be worthwhile to add some ginger to your diet. Ginger is not only great for reducing feelings of nausea, but it can help improve digestion, beat bloating and reduce gas. In addition to this, ginger is high in antioxidants and is good for boosting the immune system. To give your digestion a helping hand, try sipping on ginger tea or adding some freshly grated ginger to a fruit or vegetable juice.

Beetroot

For those needing a quick health-boosting shot of nutrients, you can't do much better than beetroot. Packed with magnesium, iron, and vitamin C, the vegetable has recently been hailed as a superfood due to its many reported health benefits. Not only is beetroot great for skin, hair and cholesterol levels, but it can also help support liver detoxification, making it an ultimate detox food. To enjoy its benefits, try adding raw beetroot to salads or sipping on some beetroot juice.

Green tea

While it's not technically a food, no detox plan would be complete without regular consumption of essential liquids. Fluids are essential for keeping our organs healthy and helping to flush toxins from the body, and drinking green tea is a great way of boosting your intake. Green tea is not only a good weight-loss drink, but it is extremely high in antioxidants. Research has also suggested that drinking green tea can protect the liver from diseases including fatty liver disease.

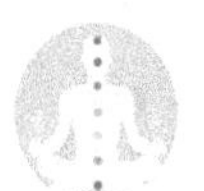

Cabbage

Many celebs have resorted to the cabbage soup diet to help them lose weight and get in shape quickly before a big event, however, cabbage is not only good for weight loss – it is also excellent detoxifying food. Like most cruciferous vegetables (including broccoli and sprouts), cabbage contains a chemical called sulforaphane, which helps the body fight against toxins. Cabbage also supplies the body with glutathione; an antioxidant that helps improve the detoxifying function of the liver.

Fresh fruit

Fresh fruits are high in vitamins, minerals, antioxidants and fibre= and are also low in calories, making them an important part of a detox diet. If you're after brighter eyes and skin, shinier hair and improved digestion, try boosting your intake of fruit and eating from a wide variety of different kinds. The good news is fruit is easy to add to your diet, so try starting your day with a fresh fruit salad or smoothie and snacking on pieces of fruit throughout the day.

Brown rice

If you want to cleanse your system and boost your health, it is a good idea to cut down on processed foods. Instead, try supplementing your diet with healthier whole grains such as brown rice, which is rich in many key detoxifying nutrients including B vitamins, magnesium, manganese and phosphorous. Brown rice is also high in fibre, which is good for cleansing the colon and rich in selenium, which can help to protect the liver as well as improving the complexion.

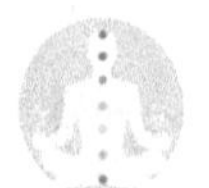

Watercress

Like most green herbs and vegetables, watercress is an excellent health booster and detox food. Firstly, watercress leaves are packed with many vital detoxifying nutrients, including several B vitamins, zinc, potassium, vitamin E and vitamin C. Secondly, watercress has natural diuretic properties, which can help to flush toxins out of the body. To reap the benefits of this nutritious food, try adding a handful of watercress to salads, soups and sandwiches.

Hibiscus Tea

When you consume a lot of sodium the body retains fluids, resulting in a paunchy belly. The flavonoids in the hibiscus plant counteract bloating by influencing how aldosterone, the hormone that regulates water and electrolytes balance, affects the body.

Bananas

By eating this fruit twice daily as a pre-meal snack can reduce belly-bloat by 50 percent Bananas have two superpowers that help slim your stomach: they increase bloat-fighting bacteria in the stomach and provide a healthy dose of potassium, which can help diminish water retention.

Blackberries

One cup of antioxidant-rich blackberries packs in 7.6 grams of fiber! Bonus: By combining the two, you trigger your gut to produce butyrate, a fatty acid that reduces fat-causing inflammation throughout your body.

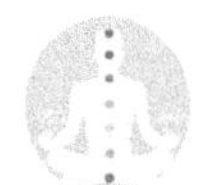

Our skin, liver, kidneys, digestive tract, and lymphatic system all have important parts to play in maintaining a balanced input and output flow. Incredibly, nature has provided us with a natural apothecary of plants that are unique enough from one another to support these various organs. From skin health to liver support, there's an herb that's right for you.

Foods That Detox the Liver

There are a handful of foods that can help detox the liver. Some of these foods include walnuts, leafy green vegetables, grapefruit and beetroot. You could even blend a handful of these ingredients together to make a detoxifying juice. Supplements like milk thistle extract, which allows you to "easily absorb a high impact antioxidant, which studies have shown to repair cell damage, particularly in the liver when caused by alcohol."

Turmeric is a great spice for detoxing the liver as well. Broccoli, cauliflower, brussel sprouts and kale are all rich in glutathione, "the antioxidant that triggers the liver-cleansing process."

Foods That Detox the Lymphatic System

"The lymphatic system moves toxins and waste products out of the body for excretion via lymph fluid, so staying hydrated is especially important. When it comes to food it is important to include apricots, cranberries, avocados and garlic in your diet if you want to help detox the lymphatic system.

Lemon and ginger can also aid in cleansing the lymphatic system

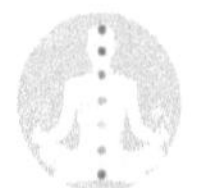

Now it is time to take a look at natural herbs that helps to detoxify our bodies, here are a list of a few.

Burdock root
Burdock is a strong tasting, bitter herb. Bitter ingredients are typically diuretics, which means they help fluids pass through the body faster. Eliminating toxins through urine.

1. Milk thistle seed
    Shanti Tea offers milk thistle seed and the leaf, and you could certainly do a mixture of both. The seed has been used for the treatment of diabetes, because of the benefits it has on the liver and gallbladder. It has shown to protect the liver from damage, and aid in the liver's glucose metabolism, lowering blood sugar. Since the liver is the bodies best detoxification organ, any ingredient which helps the liver helps detoxification overall.

2. Stinging Nettle
    Nettle leaf has a mild, sweet, slightly grassy flavour. It is great in a tea, but it can also be steamed and added to salads and soups. Be careful, dried nettle leaf will still have little stinging hairs in it!

    Nettle leaf is high in iron and vitamin C. It helps the kidneys to eliminate waste, and it supports various processes of detoxification in the liver.

3. Dandelion
    Dandelion is another mildly flavoured herb. You can buy fresh dandelion greens at many supermarkets, or look at

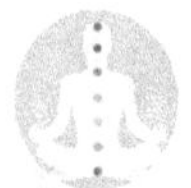

your backyard in the summer and spring. The entire plant is edible, flowers, shoots, roots and leaves. Dandelion root offers more diuretic action than the rest of the plant does.

4. Spirulina
    Rich in antioxidants, chlorophyll, protein, iron, B-vitamins, calcium and other essential nutrients, spirulina is an excellent addition to your regular diet. It has a really strong aroma and flavour, so we recommend adding it to a smoothie instead of drinking it straight. Don't infuse into hot water and risk the damage of nutrients that may be caused by adding heat to spirulina.

5. Turmeric root
    Turmeric is anti-inflammatory and contains high levels of antioxidants. The active ingredient is curcumin, which stimulates the flow of bile from the gallbladder. Bile is essential to flush out harmful toxins. Make sure to consume turmeric with black pepper because black pepper helps to activate curcumin and release many healthful benefits of turmeric root. Shanti Tea also offers cut turmeric pieces, excellent for using to create your own blends or try our anti-inflammatory blend called Vitality.

6. Green tea
    Green tea is a metabolic booster, full of antioxidants, and a diuretic. It helps all sorts of bodily functions and is great for detoxification.

7. Red clover
    Aids in blood purification and also helps to stimulate bile production, red clover has the ability to remove heavy

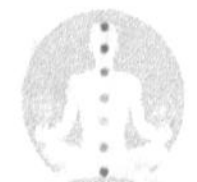

metals and chemical toxins from the body. Red clover is also a source of vitamins and minerals, such as vitamins A, C, B, magnesium, calcium, iron and phosphorous.

8. Ginger root

We love ginger. Not only does it taste great and add flavour to sweet and savoury foods and beverages, it also aids in digestion. Compounds called "gingerols" are stimulants, and help to speed the movement of food through the digestive system.

9. Mullein leaf

Mullein is an expectorant, meaning that it makes you cough. This herb is often used for a lung detox because coughing helps to clear the lungs. We especially recommend mullein for those who have recently quit smoking to help clear tar from the lungs. Studies have shown that mullein can help to expel bacteria and parasites.

Not All Water Is Good Water

Estrogen is present in our foods and in the plastics from the bottles of our drinks.

BPA is an endocrine disrupter and is known as a synthetic estrogen or a Zeno estrogen.

Companies that manufacture BPA free bottle created BPS bottles which are more dangerous than BPA. BPS was also shown to be more toxic to the reproductive system than BPA and was shown to hormonally promote certain breast cancers at the same rate as BPA

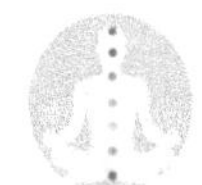

The allowed amount of atrizine in our drinking water is 3,000 nanograms

What is Atrizine ?
Atrizine is a herbicide that was used on crops in the Midwest and around the world. Atrizine disrupts the sexual development of frogs by lowering testosterone levels, they produce less sperm, and even change their mating habits by choosing males over females emasculating three-quarters of them and turning one in 10 into females.

If they are able to do this with frogs do you not think that they are capable of doing this to humans?

Scientists have now completed a draft sequence of the frog Xenopus tropicalis and found that the amphibian's genome contains remarkable similarities to those of the human genome.

You should began to wonder why so many states have legalized marijuana and ask yourself in order for it to be grown are they required to use pesticides ?

Higher estrogen levels affect women by way of them getting breast cancer, cervical cancer, fibroids etc.

Higher Estrogen in men causes testosterone levels to decrease exponentially, loss of hair, gaining weight with the inability to gain muscle etc.

I would suggest finding well water and springs that have natural water.

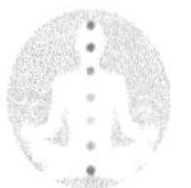

Being properly hydrated isn't about drinking water but it's more so about the minerals and electrolytes that are in the water. Melons are one of the best sources of hydration other than cucumbers.

Spring Water!

Drinking plenty of spring water a day is essential to making this alkaline diet work. Dr. Sebi suggests drinking a gallon of spring water a day, and health organizations suggest around the same amount.

The adult body consists of 70% water. All of the body's metabolic functions need adequate amounts of water to function properly. Water removes waste from the body, cushions the joints and organs, and assists in the absorption of nutrients.

Diuretics can increase urination to remove toxins from the body. You must replace the water to support the healthy functioning of the body.

Spring water is a natural alkaline water and it best supports the hydration and natural ratio of electrolytes in the body.

I strongly recommend avoiding hybrid foods (plants and their fruits made by unnaturally cross-pollinating two or more plants) because they change the genetic structure, electrical composition, and pH balance to its detriment.

One such food is garlic, a plant food we are accustomed to eating but is not the best food to consume.

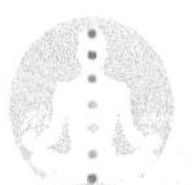

Detoxing the correct way should give you more energy, better skin, increased mental clarity and improved sleep.

The foods that we have been eating is causing catastrophic damage to our DNA but luckily for us The Source (The All) provides everything that we need in nature by way of seed bearing fruit, organic vegetables and natural herbs.

DNA is repaired when you eat foods that contain folate or folic acid. Some doctors recommend pregnant women to take folic acid because it helps build the child's brain during pregnancy. (The Fig (Black Mission Fig)is a good source of folic acid)

Eating the right foods will keep you healthy, both physically and mentally

Put the right things into the body like sea moss with bladderwrack. I speak on this because sea moss have 92 minerals out of 108 minerals that out bodies require.

Learning to fast
The fact that fasting is the cure for 90 percent of our illnesses is known by medical scientists. But, they do not teach you that.

What does the Quran say about fasting?

Al-Baqarah 2:183)
O believers! Fasting is prescribed for you—as it was for those before you1—so perhaps you will become mindful ˹of Allah˺.

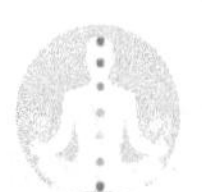

Arabic Translation

يَـٰٓأَيُّهَا ٱلَّذِينَ ءَامَنُوا۟ كُتِبَ عَلَيْكُمُ ٱلصِّيَامُ كَمَا كُتِبَ عَلَى ٱلَّذِينَ مِن قَبْلِكُمْ لَعَلَّكُمْ تَتَّقُونَ ١٨٣

Al-Baqarah 2:184)

Fast a˹ prescribed number of days.1 But whoever of you is ill or on a journey, then ˹let them fast˺ an equal number of days ˹after Ramaḍân˺. For those who can only fast with extreme difficulty,2 compensation can be made by feeding a needy person ˹for every day not fasted˺. But whoever volunteers to give more, it is better for them. And to fast is better for you, if only you knew.

Arabic Translation

أَيَّامًا مَّعْدُودَٰتٍ ۚ فَمَن كَانَ مِنكُم مَّرِيضًا أَوْ عَلَىٰ سَفَرٍ فَعِدَّةٌ مِّنْ أَيَّامٍ أُخَرَ ۚ وَعَلَى ٱلَّذِينَ يُطِيقُونَهُ فِدْيَةٌ طَعَامُ مِسْكِينٍ ۖ فَمَن تَطَوَّعَ خَيْرًا فَهُوَ خَيْرٌ لَّهُ ۚ وَأَن تَصُومُوا۟ خَيْرٌ لَّكُمْ ۖ إِن كُنتُمْ تَعْلَمُونَ ١٨٤

Al-Baqarah 2:185)

Ramaḍân is the month in which the Quran was revealed as a guide for humanity with clear proofs of guidance and the standard ˹to distinguish between right and wrong˺. So whoever is present this month, let them fast. But whoever is ill or on a journey, then ˹let them fast˺ an equal number of days ˹after Ramaḍân˺. Allah intends ease for you, not hardship, so that you may complete the prescribed period and proclaim the greatness of Allah for guiding you, and perhaps you will be grateful.

Arabic Translation

شَهْرُ رَمَضَانَ ٱلَّذِىٓ أُنزِلَ فِيهِ ٱلْقُرْءَانُ هُدًى لِّلنَّاسِ وَبَيِّنَـٰتٍ مِّنَ ٱلْهُدَىٰ وَٱلْفُرْقَانِ ۚ فَمَن شَهِدَ مِنكُمُ ٱلشَّهْرَ فَلْيَصُمْهُ ۖ وَمَن كَانَ مَرِيضًا أَوْ عَلَىٰ سَفَرٍ فَعِدَّةٌ مِّنْ أَيَّامٍ أُخَرَ ۗ يُرِيدُ ٱللَّهُ بِكُمُ ٱلْيُسْرَ وَلَا يُرِيدُ بِكُمُ ٱلْعُسْرَ وَلِتُكْمِلُوا۟ ٱلْعِدَّةَ وَلِتُكَبِّرُوا۟ ٱللَّهَ عَلَىٰ مَا هَدَىٰكُمْ وَلَعَلَّكُمْ تَشْكُرُونَ ١٨٥

Fasting in Arabic

صيام

siam

What does the Bible say about fasting?

Deuteronomy 9:18-19

Then I lay prostrate before the Lord as before, forty days and forty nights; I neither ate bread nor drank water because of all the sin you had committed, provoking the Lord by doing what was evil in his sight. 19 For I was afraid that the anger that the Lord bore against you was so fierce that he would destroy you. But the Lord listened to me that time also.

Exodus 34:28

28 He was there with the Lord forty days and forty nights; he neither ate bread nor drank water. And he wrote on the tablets the words of the covenant, the Ten Commandments.

Psalm 35:13

But as for me, when they were sick, I wore sackcloth; I afflicted myself with fasting.I prayed with head bowed on my bosom

Psalm 69:10

When I humbled my soul with fasting,[a] they insulted me for doing so.

Ezra 8:21

Fasting and Prayer for Protection

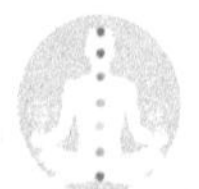

21 Then I proclaimed a fast there, at the River Ahava, that we might humble ourselves[a] before our God, to seek from him a safe journey for ourselves, our children, and all our possessions.

Matthew 6:16-18
When you fast, do not look somber as the hypocrites do, for they disfigure their faces to show others they are fasting. Truly I tell you, they have received their reward in full. But when you fast, put oil on your head and wash your face, so that it will not be obvious to others that you are fasting, but only to your Father, who is unseen; and your Father, who sees what is done in secret, will reward you.

Zechariah 7:4-5
Then the word of the Lord Almighty came to me, "Ask all the people of the land and the priests, 'When you fasted and mourned in the fifth and seventh months for the past seventy years, was it really for me that you fasted?"

Fasting cleanses the arteries and eyes; it enhances the nerves, the cognitive state and continence or temperament. Dr. Sebi talks about how it lowers high blood pressure and he often speaks about a 21-day fast.

During his very own healing process in Mexico when he fasted, he reports being calm the first 7 days and then becoming dizzy every day after the 7th day on to the 15th day. He noted how he was so dizzy that he had to crawl to the bathroom on all fours for a whole week on his knees and hands; explaining how he couldn't stand up because everything seemed to be moving. On the 16th day he experiences a peace that he is

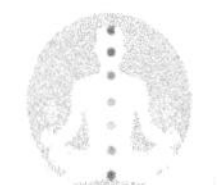

unable to remember ever experiencing before. He noticed that he was no longer wheezing on the 27th day.

- Diabetes ~ Gone
- impotency ~ Gone
- Asthma ~ Gone

Studies discovered that intermittent fasting boosts working memory in animals and verbal memory in adult humans. Heart health. Intermittent fasting improved blood pressure and resting heart rates as well as other heart-related measurements.

When we fast, our bodies run on stored energy. Initially, that energy comes from glycogen, the stored form of glucose found in the liver and the muscles. But once we've fasted for some time, the liver runs out of glycogen and switches to producing chemicals called ketone bodies from metabolizing fat.

Most would like to believe that fasting is more about food but it is about focus and it can be used as a process to heal the body. Fasting is not so much about saying no to the body but more about saying yes to the Spirit.

IMPOTENCE OR ERECTION DISFUNCTION

Dr. Sebi addresses how all the fat that we have been eating over the years begins to clog the penis and prostate gland. Being impotent at age 30, he says he had an erection on his 29th day of fasting. Fasting gives the body the opportunity to drain itself of the buildup of calcification, cholesterol, triglycerides and the rest.

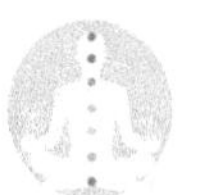

The orifice of the penis is spongy; it needs blood to flow but the orifices are clogged. Fasting will help it to drain out.

ASTHMA
Dr. Sebi reports how his asthma cleared up due to fasting.

ARTHRITIS
Dr. Sebi reports how he put his mother on a 52 day fast; consuming only water and his compounds. Afterward, her arthritis was gone and she was able to lift her arms above her head.

SIMPLE RULES of starting Intermittent fasting -"IF"for fat loss:

It takes time to adapt to the fasting/feeding schedule.

Start with a longer feeding window. Gradually work up to a longer fasting period.

No food (calories) during the fast.

Don't push your workouts to extremes, especially in the beginning. Go intense after eating, or skip "IF" on the day you want to do an extreme workout.

Don't gorge when feeding. Do not overeat. Eat slowly to aid digestion. Spread meals out throughout the feeding window.

Avoid junk food and poor eating habits. "IF" will not negate the effects of these "foods." Get your nutrition from whole, nutritious, nutrient dense, high-quality foods.

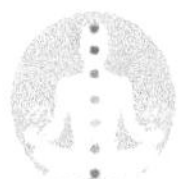

Stay hydrated. Drink lots of water.

The task where healing must be accomplished is found in the pH balance in the body's blood. Immunology reveals that getting sick, acquiring diseases and bad microbes are due to a deficiency in the body which affects the immune system. If the pH of the body is acidic, then it will strip the body of it's mineral nutrients and deprived the body's ability to have a strong immune system.

Keep in mind that during some healing or cleansing processes, you will need to get more rest than usual. Depending on your situation, you may need to prepare to endure what is referred to as the healing crisis; which in short means to expect things to get worse before they get better. This has a lot to do with why Dr. Sebi uses the terminology of "reversing disease," because during the healing process the body is known to re-visit each kind of pain, skin rash or disease that it experienced prior to the healing; all depending on how long the healing process is. Dr. Sebi has addressed at least eight things regarding the method of boosting the immune system.

THE METHOD
1. Fasting
2. Alkaline herbal Compounds
3. A Gallon of Water a Day
4. Exercise
5. Refrain from consuming detrimental foods
6. Eat according to a list of foods that Dr. Sebi has recommended.
7. Sleep (be kind to your body and get some rest)
8. Usha Village (or stress

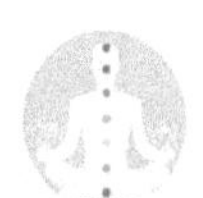

The late elder Dick Gregory made a reference about fasting "If you took a comb and combed your hair which hair would probably come out on the comb the weak ones or the strong ones ? The body will respond to the weak cells the same way when you heal yourself through fasting

So we must overstand that fasting is very much essential to our spiritual health and physical wellbeing

When to eat

Even thought Muslims observe a strict daily fast from dawn until sunset during Ramadan I must say that when you are not fast the most important time to eat is in the morning. As they say Breakfast (when you break fast) is the most important meal of the day and I will explain why.

Breakfast breaks the overnight fasting period. It replenishes your supply of glucose to boost your energy levels and alertness, while also providing other essential nutrients required for good health.

We are Sun people, the sun is key to our existence so the sun plays a major in healing us also. Another reason it is important to eat in the morning is because during daylight the solar energy from the sun energizes our body to help burn off the foods we consume.

I my opinion Dr. Sebi was not just a herbalist but a scientist when it came to herbs and the human body. His mission and vision was to open healing centers in all the major cities and start healing people for free.

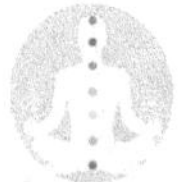

The family members of Dr.Sebi have opened a healing village
In the state of Georgia

USHA Healing Family

USA suite 500, 5071 Peachtree Blvd,
Chamblee, GA 30341

Note: I am not a doctor and can only tell you what is working for me. This guide is working for me!)

The foods that we eat have us thinking and acting out of our mind I say this because of the parasite in the food that controls our behavior, the damage of our DNA caused by the Neurotoxins ,chemicals, additives and preservatives that are put in our foods and also because of the acidic foods that we consume block and corrode our neurons.

It is time that we began to repair the damage and start the healing process. We have learned the foods that are essential for healing the body but now it is time to repair the mind.

Brain Food
Goji berries
Blue berries
Strawberries
Black berries
Pimento (allspice) berry
Chaste (bites) berries

Berries are very high in antioxidants and are oxygenators which is what the brain needs to get the melanin neurotransmitters

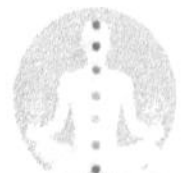

and the dendrites connected to the left side and the right side of the brain. The brain needs oxygen and can get it through iron phosphate going through the blood.

Antioxidants

An antioxidant is a compound that inhibits oxidation. Oxidation is a chemical reaction that can produce chain reactions and free radicals, and therefore has the potential of doing damage to the body's cells.

Antioxidants have the potential to delay various forms of cognitive decline, like memory loss. This is all related to oxidative stress, too, which can contribute to Alzheimer's disease and other forms of memory loss and decline in cognitive function.

The major antioxidants sources are vitamin C, vitamin E, beta-carotene, and other related carotenoids, along with the minerals selenium and manganese.

Benefits of Antioxidants

They reduce oxidative stress.

They support disease prevention.

They support eye health.

They aid in brain function.

They can contribute to mental health improvements.

They can reduce inflammation

They support healthy aging processes.

Herbs That Are Good For The Memory

kalawalla herb (helps if someone is suffering from Dementia and Alzheimer's)

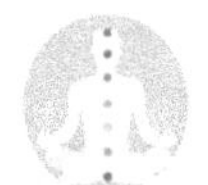

Granny back bone bark
Capadulla
Chaney Root
sarsaparilla root
Monkey Ladder

Eat But Don't Pig Out

I CAN ONLY HELP YOU IF YOU ARE WILLING TO HELP YOURSELF

 I want you to overstand how harmful our eating habits are to our health and wellbeing. I feel that it is my responsibility to inform on the history of the pig and it's purpose. I want you to see the scheme of how porky the pig is incorporated into every single thing that we consume and this is not by chance. We must learn to detox from consuming poisons and toxins and learn to heal ourselves through fasting and prayer . We also must learn to put the right things into our bodies in order to think and function properly. We must gain a higher sense of self through strict discipline of what, how and when we eat. We have to get back to divinity.

Eat But Don't Pig Out
The Right way to eat and heal your body

I CAN ONLY HELP YOU IF YOU ARE WILLING TO HELP YOURSELF

I hope that you have been following me this far because this is a very important journey and we must overstand that it a

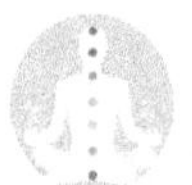

matter of life, mental health and physical health what we put into our bodies. When we start thinking with our right mind we will overstand that health is true wealth and the first part of being wealth is through health.

We must learn to make our way back to divinity starting with the way we eat and I say this because what we eat controls how we think and how our bodies function.

As Tupac said in one of his most remembered songs "Changes" We had to change the way we live, change the way we eat and change the way we treat each other.

I wrote this book because I truly care for my people and I want to be an influence on us changing our lives for the better we must learn to eat correctly in order for us to live healthy and prosperous lives.

In conclusion it is my mission to inform my people that the Hazardous and poisonous so called foods that we consume mainly pork is detrimental to our health and growth. With this book you will learn what the Most High says about which foods to eat and which foods to not eat through scriptures, you will learn which foods not to eat and why you shouldn't be consuming them, which foods that make you age, you will be informed on which foods and herbs to eat that detoxify your body so that you can cleanse your organs of any toxins and impurities and last but not least you will learn the best times to eat and when not to eat through fasting.

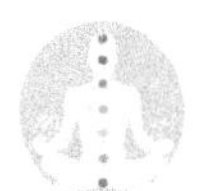

If you have made a donation to receive this book I would like to say thank you and you are greatly appreciated. The journey does not end here there will be more books on the way. I am working on producing more informative content so please add my social media like and share, again you are greatly appreciated.

I CAN ONLY HELP YOU IF YOU ARE
WILLING TO HELP YOURSELF

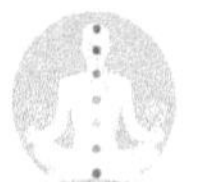

Donations are welcome and can be sent to
Light Walker LLC at P.O. 81581
Athens GA 30608